THE

SEX

CHRONICLES

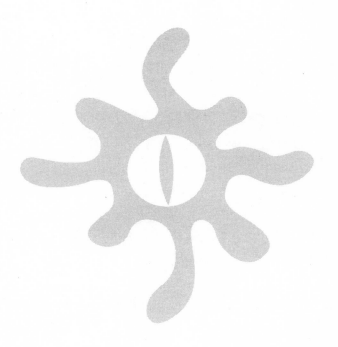

Publisher: W. Quay Hays
Editorial Director: Peter L. Hoffman
Editor: Steve Baeck
Production Director: Trudihope Schlomowitz
Prepress Manager: Bill Castillo
Copyeditor: Mark Lamana

For information:

General Publishing Group, Inc.
2701 Ocean Park Boulevard, Suite 140
Santa Monica, CA 90405

Library of Congress Cataloging-in-Publication Data

Rancier, Lance.
    The sex chronicles : Strange-but-true tales from
around the world / by Lance Rancier.
       p.   cm.
    ISBN 1-57544-081-4
    1. Sex—Miscellanea. 2. Sex—Anecdotes. I. Title.
HQ25.R34 1998
306.7—dc21   98-4868
                                          CIP

Printed in the USA
by Royal Book Manufacturing
10 9 8 7 6 5 4 3 2 1

Jacket Design: Robert Avellan
Cover photo © Larry Fink

General Publishing Group
Los Angeles

T H E

SEX

CHRONICLES

Strange-But-True

TALES

*From Around
the World*

BY LANCE RANCIER

GENERAL
PUBLISHING
GROUP, INC

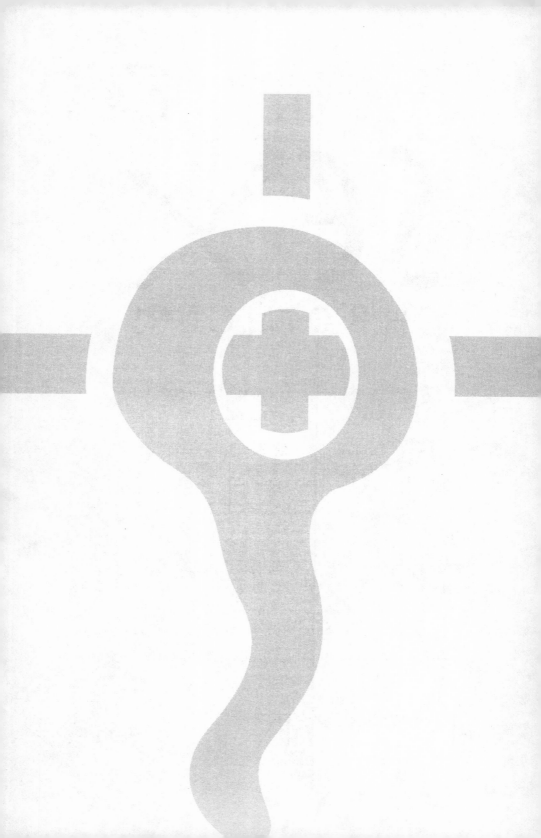

Contents

"He ceased; but left so pleasing on the ear his voice, that list'ning still they seemed to hear."

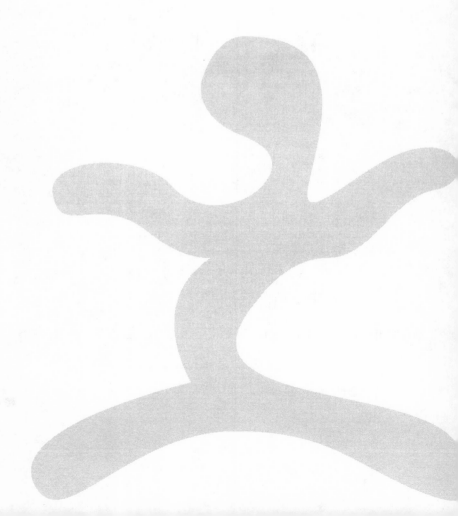

For Mom and Dad, Doug, Candace and Lisa—
for all your love and support.
And for Nancy, who was so good to me.
Many thanks to M.R.

The author welcomes your comments and suggestions.
Please send them to the author, care of

General Publishing Group, Inc.
2701 Ocean Park Blvd., Suite 140
Santa Monica, CA 90405

Corruption, vice and laxity are the rule today. This is particularly true among our youth. Our society cannot endure, for the young men of our race are given up unto vain pleasures. They think not of the morrow. They live in folly for the day. Woe, woe to our land, the land of our fathers.

Urukagina, Sumerian ruler
2545 B.C.

You made us guilty, you, Romulus, who suckled the harsh wolf. You taught your men to rape the Sabines freely: now love does anything, and rules your Rome.

Sextus Propertius, Roman poet
1st Century B.C.

What am I to call you? You haven't yet proved yourselves men. All you wish is freedom for sensuality and excess.

Augustus Caesar, Roman emperor
1st Century A.D.

A woman's morals nowadays are as changeable as cat's eyes.

Ejima Kiseki, writer
15th Century

Listen and give ear. We are living in a day of unrestrained license. It is time to call a halt.

Li Yu, Chinese writer
1657

People do not have passions any more. Debauchery and false love are rife. I prophesize that lack of affection and incapacity to feel will lead this country to perdition.

Marquis d'Argenson, French nobleman
1715

The times in which we live are in no danger of adopting a system of romantic virtue. The present generation have contrived to bring down that idle, youthful, unprofitable passion. The levity of dissipation, vanity of parade, and the fury of gaming have concurred to cure completely the tendency to mutual fondness.

James Fordyce, English writer
1766

Somebody was calculating recently the length of time to be hoped for, before, at the present rate, all the world would go mad. At the present rate of increase the time is surely within easy calculation....

Sylvanus Stall, American doctor/writer
1897

In olden days a glimpse of stocking, Was looked on as something shocking, Now heaven knows, Anything goes.

Cole Porter, American songwriter, from "Anything Goes"
1934

It was the complaint of our ancestors, as it is ours, and will be that of posterity, that morality has changed, and wickedness rules, and mankind goes from bad to worse, and everything sacred is falling into disrepute. This one thing is and ever will be the same—changing its extent from time to time, like seaways which the incoming tide drives on and the ebb keeps back and constrains.

You are wrong, Lucilius, if you think that our age is peculiar for vice, luxury, desertion of moral standards, and all the other things which everyone imputes to his own time. These are the faults of mankind, not of any age. No time in history has been free of guilt.

Seneca, Roman statesman/philosopher
1st Century A.D.

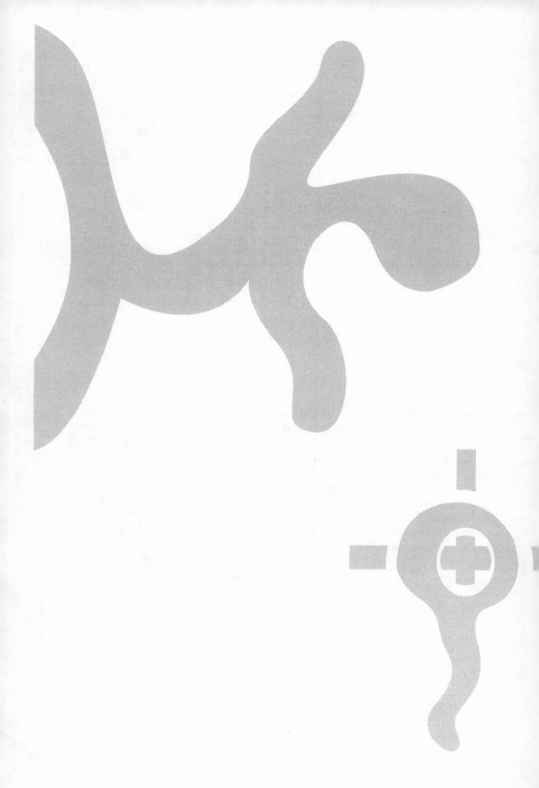

SEX AND THE LAW

Progress has often been considered dangerous to morals:

When feather beds were introduced into Argentina, they were declared illegal in the city of Buenos Aires. They were not allowed because they promoted "lascivious feelings."

Dowries have been a common part of marriage throughout the world. In some cases, the dowry was treated as a symbolic gesture, of little real value. In other cases, it was strictly enforced by law:

The Welsh of the Middle Ages had a complete set of legal dowry obligations. Marriages were not considered legal until the Amobyr, or Gobyr, was paid for the girl's virginity. The dowry was dependent on the position of the woman, whether she be a king's daughter, chief's daughter, or foreigner's daughter.

The dowry was equal to the value of the father's land. It was paid to the king or lord for the protection of females within his land. It was paid by her relatives if she was given to a man by them. If she married the man of her own choice, she herself was responsible for paying the dowry. If a girl chose to give her virginity away to a lover without being married, she was also obligated to pay the dowry herself.

The Amobyr was payable even if the girl was kidnapped—and paid by her abductor.

The incest taboo has been especially strong in China:

Family names in China had one of three sources: They came from the region of the family's ancestors, or from the town or village of their origin, or from a position held by an ancestor. For all the millions of Chinese, there were only 100 original last names. Despite the very great odds of having similar last names, couples with the same last name were, by law, forbidden to marry.

However distant their connection, Chinese couples even vaguely related were forbidden to marry. If a man, for instance, had an affair with the wife of his father's cousin three times removed, he had committed incest.

♂♀

Although the ancient Chinese had a rich erotic life, the law came down hard on those who were too explicit:

The ancient Chinese used exotic terms to describe the act of intercourse and the organs used. These romantic names were used because the Chinese people thought the proper names were too "rude" to use. If a writer used these crude terms for sex and sexual parts, he was beheaded.

♂♀

There have been many extremes in the way different cultures dealt with adultery. Some have been very forgiving, others were very severe:

If a Pasema man found his wife committing adultery in his own home, he was legally allowed to kill his wife's sexual partner then and there.

However, if the husband came across the couple anywhere else, he was not allowed to get his revenge by killing the man, even if the husband caught the couple having sex.

Among the North American Inuit of the far north, a husband who discovered the unfaithfulness of his wife might feel obligated to save his honor by killing his wife's lover. If he didn't, the wrong could be cleared another way: The husband and his wife's lover had a "singing duel."

♂♀

For a very long time, and until very recently in some places, adultery was a crime for which only the woman was punished:

The Sumerian Law of 1100 B.C. treated adultery not as a crime of morals, but as a crime of property—the husband's property. The husband was allowed his sexual freedom, but the woman of the time had to stay faithful to her husband or be punished.

Women's economic dependence on men has often put them at a great disadvantage:

In New England in the 17th century, a man and a woman convicted of adultery were publicly humiliated. They were forced to get down on their hands and knees in front of their village and beg for forgiveness.

After this, they had to strip nude to the waist, and be whipped. They could avoid the whipping, however, by paying a fine. Men usually paid the fine to escape the pain and humiliation of being thrashed.

Women, rarely having money of their own, almost always had to face their neighbors half nude, and be whipped.

The 11th-century king Canute established a severe penalty for adultery. The woman's lover was sent out of the country and never allowed to return. The woman, as her punishment, had her ears and nose cut off.

A great number of cultures have considered the breaking of adultery laws as punishable only by death:

The ancient Aztecs of the Valley of Mexico sentenced men and women guilty of adultery, to have their heads crushed between two huge stones.

Penance for adultery could last a long time:

The Celtic king, King Edgar, made sure that the sin of adultery was not soon forgiven or forgotten. Adulterers and adulteresses paid for their sexual indulgence by having to live on bread and water three days a week, for seven years.

Adultery on the part of females has been considered whoring, and has often been punished that way:

In ancient Sumeria, a married man's wife was, basically, the one who was punished when her husband was caught having sex with a single woman. The husband was forced by law to marry his lover. The completely innocent first wife was given to her husband's lover's father to be used as his own prostitute.

The ancient Roman woman who was guilty of committing adultery paid heavily for her mistake. For a full day after she was found guilty, she was forced to sexually satisfy any and all men who wanted to have sex with her. A lottery was held to see who her first sexual partner would be.

In some instances, prostitutes have had more sexual rights than wives:

In 17th-century England, a whore could bring charges against a man for rape. The woman, however, who was a wife, mistress, or concubine to a man who had forced her to have sex, had no legal right to claim rape. All male lovers' sexual advances were considered legally proper.

In a vast number of cultures, punishment for adultery has been dealt out strictly to restore the honor of a wronged partner—usually the man. In some cases, soothing the jealousy has gone to extremes:

In East Africa, the Wadshaggas punished the man who committed adultery with another man's wife by forcing him to pay a fine to the offended husband. As someone who had also publicly embarrassed the husband, the person who had revealed the wife's affair had to pay a fine of the same amount.

The Tungu man who learned of his wife's cheating on him was allowed to kill his wife's lover. Since his pride was hurt also by the person who exposed the affair, he was also entitled to kill the messenger.

At certain times in history, rape had very far-reaching results:

It was the law of the Athelstan king in the 10th century that a man who raped a virgin from a powerful family was first castrated, and then killed. The punishment did not stop there, however. The offender had punishment also inflicted upon his dog and horse. The law was that their "...scrotum and tail...shall be cut off as close as possible to the buttocks."

In ancient Peru, a man who committed adultery, or even attempted to seduce one of the many wives or concubines of the Inca, was disposed of quickly. The couple were executed together by being burned alive.

As well, all the man's near relatives, parents, wives, children and others were killed. The people of the man's town or village were driven away from their homes, and the houses and trees were destroyed. Then salt was spread over the ground of the ghost town, so that nothing would grow.

The most common style of ancient law was that of revenge, or "An eye for an eye, a tooth for a tooth":

In ancient Assyria, the Lex Talionis dealt out justice through revenge.

A virgin who had been sexually violated by a married man had the injury "righted" by having her father rape the rapist's wife.

ℰ

Primitive cultures have often treated sexual crimes very harshly:

In the 1500s, the Colombian Amani of the Central Cordillera region punished adulterers this way: The man was simply killed. His female partner was imprisoned in a dark room. Every man in the village who wanted to have sex with her did so. Then she was killed. Both of the lovers' bodies were then publicly displayed and left to rot.

The Pathans made examples of adulterers and adulteresses by making them the objects of slow and painful deaths. The male was staked out in the hot sun, and then hot pepper stalks were thrust up his anus. Sharp and knobby thorns were pushed into his penis. Then he was kicked in the testicles until he was dead.

The female, for her part, was tied to a stake, her legs spread wide apart around a quickly growing plant. The plant grew inside her vagina until it painfully killed her.

ℰ

The law has always been a matter of judgment. Sometimes the lack of information or prejudice of the times affected these judgments:

In Wales during the Middle Ages, if the husband of a new bride suspected that his wife had not come to the wedding night with her virginity, he called the marriage guests together the next morning. The bride was obligated to swear an oath that she had come to the marriage a virgin. The oath was enough to convince, if she was 12 years old or younger. If she was older, she needed at least five character witnesses. If she could not deny the charge, she was stripped nude to the hips. A three-year-old bull was brought in to the trial. To collect the three-year-old bull as payment for having given up her virginity, and then having been deserted by her lover, the woman had to undergo a test. The bull's tail was shaved and greased, and the woman grabbed the tail. If she could hold on to it, she kept it as payment for her shame. If not, all she was allowed to keep was the grease on her hands.

ℰ

In 17th-century England, sexual contact with a woman without her consent was considered rape. However, "if the woman at the time of the supposed rape, do conceive with child, by the ravisher, this is no rape, for a woman cannot conceive with child except she do consent."

Just as a woman has been obligated to pay the consequences of pregnancy with childbirth, so has she often born the full legal responsibility for the results of the sexual connection:

In Virginia in the 1600s, a man who forced himself on his female servant was guiltless. Very often it was the poor servant girl who paid for her employer's weakness. If a servant became pregnant as a result of her master's misconduct, the church wardens took care of her. However, to pay for her trouble, the girl had to work for two years, with her pay going back to the church.

♂♀

Adultery has typically been the most severely punished sexual deviation, because it undermined the family unit. In some societies, the family unit was not as important as class distinction:

In India, the Baiswars of Mirzapur considered adultery a less serious offense than eating with another person who was not of the same caste, or class.

♂♀

An uneasy truce has often existed between sexual deviants and the community:

In the 1870s, Paris, France, had certain public areas reserved for sodomists. The area was quite strictly policed, and there were quality standards for the catamites. The boys who made their living there were divided into three classes. First, there were the healthy, fresh youths. Second were the boys without testicles, but still with sexual powers. The third and lowest class consisted of those who could not achieve an erection. This last class was tested to make sure that erection was impossible. They lay on a mattress with the bottom open and were vigorously and consistently manipulated by two whores. Another prostitute whipped their sexual parts with stinging-needles. This procedure was followed for 15 minutes. Then long red peppers were inserted into their anuses. The stinging-needles by this time had formed blisters, and mustard was spread over them. If the catamites passed this test and no erection was achieved, they were hired out to men only as passive partners, at one-third the standard price.

♂♀

In 1443 the Venice town council passed a law that made it a crime for a male to dress up as a female and walk the streets. This was called "unfair competition."

Sodomy was a very common practice in 15th-century Venice. Many laws were passed to try to curb this practice. One of these laws was passed in 1480 and made it illegal for whores to dress as men and capitalize on this sexual preference.

In the 17th century in Italy, Lodovico Maria Sinistrari required that all lesbians be examined. Any woman who had a clitoris any larger than the norm was dealt with harshly. The woman with an enlarged clitoris was considered capable of committing sodomy on her fellow women, and put to death.

In 16th-century Geneva, the courts decided that they must deal with the "crime" of lesbianism. While cases of male homosexuality were described in a certain amount of detail, it was decided that female homosexual acts could not—and nothing whatever was said of the activities. Germain Colladron explained: "A crime so horrible and against nature is so detestable, and because of the horror of it, it cannot be named."

At times, prostitution has been not only legal, but encouraged by the civil authority:

In 1439, in Bourg-en-Bresse, France, the community subsidized the building of a large brothel. This was not uncommon. The municipality of Villefranche-sur-Saone bought the local whorehouse in 1440, and St. Flour opened one of their own in the 1440s.

In Treviso, Italy, in the mid-16th century, a woman guilty of lesbianism was stripped naked and tied to a stake located in the Street of Locusts. She stood there under guard for one day and one night, then was taken outside the city and burned alive.

Where prostitution was tolerated, whores were often required by law to distinguish themselves from the general population:

In ancient Rome in 370 A.D., a law was passed requiring that harlots dye their hair blond. This system was the formalization of a tradition begun many years before. This was the most obvious way of distinguishing fallen women from others, as the Mediterranean women were brunette and olive-skinned. It is also believed that it was a continuance from the practice of King Solomon, who kidnapped fair-skinned, blond women for their "novelty value."

An unusual legal punishment utilized the "mother-in-law taboo," which was very common in many primitive cultures:

The penalty for a man who lied under oath in Papua: He was forced to shake hands with his mother-in-law.

In general, laws have restricted women from having property rights, often because women themselves were considered their husband's property. This is not universally true, however:

In ancient Wales, a woman was allowed property rights not usually granted to her sisters of the times. She had as much right to separate from her husband as he had to leave her. If she misbehaved with another man or committed adultery, she could be divorced, with the husband retaining all the marital property. However, should she want to divorce him, she was entitled to the property if she proved that he had leprosy, was impotent, or had very bad breath.

Jealous restriction of contact with another person's mate has been taken to some extremes:

The Pantiaak Malays killed the man who saved a drowning woman, unless she was related to him.

Divorce could be a very easy procedure, often easier than getting married:

Under Moslem law, a divorce was as simple as the husband saying "I divorce thee."
He could divorce the same woman twice this way. If, after divorcing her twice, he changed his mind and desired her back, he was required to have her married and then divorced.
Often a Mustehhel or Mohellil ("intermediary") was used. The mustehhel was usually a very young (about seven years old) black slave boy. The woman married him, slept with him, and then divorced him. It was only then that her previous husband could remarry her.

Some societies have made it nearly impossible to legally dissolve a marriage:

In the late 17th century in England, a legal civil divorce could be secured only by first proving spotlessness of character, then obtaining a separation from the ecclesiastical courts. Once this was satisfied, a divorce could be granted only by a Special Act of Parliament.
This, of course, cost thousands of pounds, which permitted only the very wealthy to apply for a divorce. In addition, the only grounds by which a man could secure a divorce was adultery.
Worse for the woman was that she could apply for a divorce only if she could prove incestuous and adulterous intercourse by her husband. In nearly 200 years, only about 300 divorces were granted.

It has been possible in some societies to legally change sex—in manner, anyway. However, the laws of the land still applied to these transvestites:

In the western Balkans, it was common to find that an only child who was female or the eldest in a family of daughters assumed the character of a boy. This was perfectly accepted by all, providing the transvestite gave up her right to be a mother. As a boy, she was considered a sworn virgin.

It was a crime if, after they had assumed their male identity, they later had intercourse with men. Should they break this law, they were dealt with severely. In Montenegro they were stoned to death, and in Northern Albania they were burned alive.

Ancient civilizations were careful to protect the capacity to reproduce. Strict laws were implemented to ensure that men's organs of reproduction were kept healthy:

The ancient Assyrians had a law against the threat of loss of a man's reproductive powers: "If a woman has crushed a man's testicle in an affray, one of her fingers shall be cut off."

A law from the book of Deuteronomy provided a harsh penalty for a woman who damaged the reproductive organs:

"When men fight with one another, and the wife of the one draws near to rescue her husband from the hand who is beating him, and puts out her hand and seizes him by the private parts, then you shall cut off her hand."

When a woman was wronged by a man's organ, she was obligated to reacquaint herself with it while testifying against him:

The King of Wales in the 10th century, Howel Dda, passed an interesting piece of legislation. A woman, in swearing her complaint against her attacker, went through an unusual ritual. "She must...place her right hand upon the relics of the saints, and her left hand upon the virile member of the accused."

The family unit and pairing of men and women has been one of the more structured of legal functions. Preservation and promotion of the household was a main preoccupation of lawmakers of nearly all civilizations:

In Dardistan and Astar, to drink raw milk with a woman automatically engaged her to the man sharing the drink with her.

A fatherless household was socially undesirable, and laws were made to lessen its likelihood. The widespread custom that obligated a man to marry his dead brother's wife was known as Levirate. It comes from the latin *Levir*, or "brother-in-law":

It was forbidden amongst the Zulus for two sisters to be married at the same time. This was perhaps in the event of the death of one of the sisters. The single sibling was obligated to replace her dead sister as wife in her widowed brother-in-law's household.

The Hungarian man who married two women and was found out, was not obliged to give one of the women up. Instead, his punishment was to live with both women under the same roof.

Under seventh-century Kretan law, a property-holding widow was legally obligated to remarry. Further, she had no choice in who she married: Once widowed, she must marry her father's brother. If the uncle on the father's side was dead, she had to marry a cousin. This selection continued until a male on her father's side could be paired off with her.

In northwestern India, among the Bharia of Juhbulpore and the Khapariya, if a man caught his wife committing adultery, he could not divorce her. However, he could secure a divorce if he caught her and warned her three times. It was only after the third incident that he could be legally divorced.

In some instances of law, what was considered legal may not have always been considered fair:

The Courts of Love, which settled affairs of the heart in medieval Europe, were far more compassionate than the laws of the civil courts. Civil law allowed a man to thrash his wife "to a reasonable extent." The Courts of Love refused to allow husbands to strike their wives at all.

In the state of Virginia, in 1791, a new law was passed concerning adultery. While the punishment for adultery was a steep fine or public flogging, a much harsher punishment was put forward for interracial intercourse.

Any white person caught having sex with a mulatto (part white, part black person), "Negro" or Indian was banished from the colony.

The law has always favored the interests of the locality over foreign freedoms, especially where immigration is concerned:

The ancient Nordic peoples castrated foreign wanderers entering their countries. This was to prevent their fathering a child and then leaving the mother. The Gragas, the oldest Icelandic code of law, allowed a wandering man to be castrated without punishment upon those who performed the surgery. Even in the event of his death, the castrators were blameless, protected under the law.

The delicate subjects of sex and love became public at one time, to be openly disputed in front of impartial arbiters:

The Countess of Champagne, with a jury of 60 other women, presided over a case in the Courts of Love in France during the Middle Ages. A typical case involved a messenger of love-notes who took a fancy to the woman receiving the love-notes and proceeded to attempt to win her for himself. His punishment was banishment from the company of the honest persons, including banishment from the social event of the day—tournaments.

Pagan and tribal societies have often had surprisingly comprehensive laws concerning marriage and divorce:

In pagan Ireland, the Brehom Laws listed seven grounds on which women could apply for divorce. She could part from a husband who had disfigured her through violence. A woman had grounds for divorce if the husband had replaced her with another woman. If he had seduced her by means of a magic potion while courting, she could leave him. A wife could leave her husband if he withheld his services in bed "so that he prefers to lie with servant boys when it is not necessary"; also, if she could not receive her pleasure by his performance in bed. She could also separate from a husband who had circulated malicious gossip about her, or who said things about her to the neighbors, which made her the laughingstock.

Homosexuals in America in the 1880s had very poor legal status:

The 19th-century American courts regarded homosexuals as little more than idiots or mentally ill degenerates, and classified homosexuals as one of the many kinds of the criminally insane.

Persecution of homosexuals has often been vigorous, and their sexual preference legally punishable:

In the 15th century, several Italian cities instituted "sodomy courts." Called Ufficiali di Notte, these courts were a part of Italian life for at least 70 years. Citizens were requested to drop the names of suspected sodomites in boxes. These boxes were set up in public places in the cities.

One of the more notable people accused was a certain Leonardo da Vinci. His accuser was Jacopo Saltatelli, a 17-year-old artist's model. Da Vinci proclaimed his innocence but expressed regret at having employed the boy, who, da Vinci admitted, had a "bad reputation." Da Vinci was acquitted of the charges.

There have occurred instances of legal persecution for bestiality:

In Paris in 1750, Jacques Ferron, of the suburb of the Vauvres, was charged with having unnatural relations with a she-ass. Ferron's guilt was proved, and he took his punishment the day he was hanged. The other "guilty" party, however, received a stay of execution when friends came to her rescue. The prioress of the convent at Vauvres, having known the she-ass for several years, swore a legal oath as to the purity of the animal. The prioress claimed that because of the previous decency of the beast, the ass would not have willingly participated in Ferron's escapades. The courts were convinced, and the ass escaped criminal prosecution.

Lawmakers have not always legislated to protect public morality as much as to protect their own interests:

In ancient Rome, a cult accumulated a large and vigorous following. This was the cult of Bacchanalia, one which attracted a great number of erotomaniacs. The cult started in southern Italy, spread northward and became very popular because the festivals featured violence, sex and general pandemonium. Originally, the cult was only for women, but this changed when a priestess initiated her sons into the society. The sexual anarchy increased as the congregation started consisting of both males and females. With the fear that the society was becoming too popular, the Roman senate ordered the prosecution of members, and approximately 7,000 people were tried. A great number of the accused were executed, and the others not in custody fled Rome.

In 186 B.C., the senate decreed that Bacchanalia was forbidden. This relieved the powerful men of Rome, who feared losing their power.

Roman law was concerned with the sexual status of a woman who was to be executed for her crime:

In ancient Rome, under Emperor Tiberius (42 B.C.–A.D. 37), the bodies of executed people were thrown on the Stairs of Mourning and then dragged to the Tiber River. It was law that a virgin could not be executed. Thus, the executioner was instructed to first rape a virgin offender, who was then executed.

Nearly every society has created laws to limit the spread of social diseases:

In ancient India, it was against the law for a bachelor to own a female alpaca, a camel-like creature. This animal was thought to have given its human lovers syphilis as punishment for mating with animals.

The incest taboo has often been a violent one, with severe measures to punish the lawbreakers:

The Malaysian couple who were related and found to be having sex were treated severely. They were taken to the graveyard of their relatives. A hole was dug, and the couple was tossed in and buried alive— to spend eternity together, amongst their relatives.

The ancient Cayapans of southern Ecuador did not tolerate the practice of incestuous relations. Those who broke the incest taboo were suspended over a table covered with candles and roasted to death.

Knowledge is power—especially in the case of sex:

Because the French university students of the Middle Ages were part of the intelligent elite, they were very politically useful to their kings. Because they were part of a small minority of the educated and young and strong as well, they were a king's valuable ally. For this reason, they enjoyed great freedom.

In return for their support, they had the privilege to move about freely, thieving, indulging in thuggery, and pursuing women. They were essentially above the law. The young men enjoyed every freedom with whore or innocent girl, whether she consented or not.

Laws have been primarily used to censure or regulate the incidence of intercourse. There have been instances when legislation was provided to promote it:

Early in the Chinese Han dynasty (A.D. 200–250), an emperor was dismayed by the lack of sexual activity among his people. To promote coupling, the emperor enumerated all unattached males over 30 and all single girls older than 20. These men and women were then commanded to mate with each other before the following spring. Those bashful or unpopular types who didn't succeed were given 100 lashes.

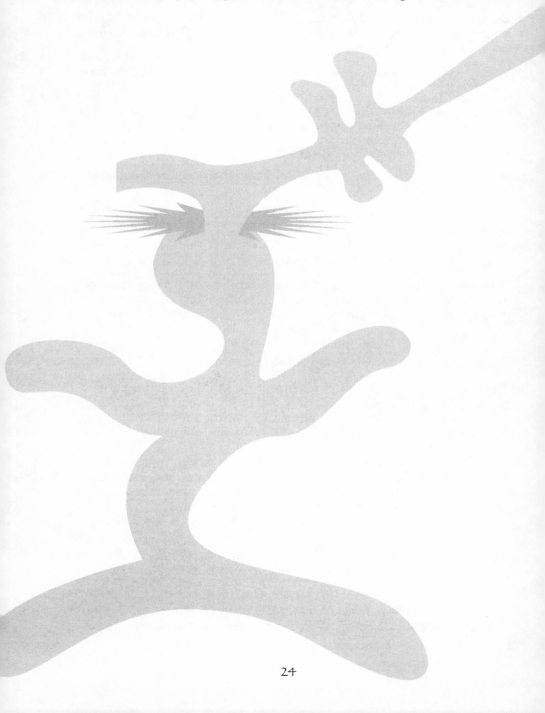

MANNERS

In Bolivia, a man could divorce his wife for having more than a few sips of wine. If she had more than this very small amount, her husband could accuse her of advertising to everyone that she was sexually loose.

In many cultures as diverse as Irish, African, Asian and ancient Roman, the mannerly woman thought nothing of exposing her breasts but was horrified at revealing her foot:

In ancient Rome, the respectable Roman woman wore a toga, or Stola, which was weighted at the bottom so as to always cover her foot. Only courtesans and nymphs celebrating erotic festivals dared exposed their feet.

In northwestern Siberia, the Yakut girls, as part of their household duties, exposed their thighs while wrapping thread around them, and they were not shy if strangers saw them doing this. It did not bother them to have men observe them topless. However, they took great care in concealing both their feet and hair from their male in-laws.

In Siberia and in eastern and central Russia, on very hot days it was common that women publicly went virtually naked, with one exception: The feet were carefully covered. The most overt sexual act among these people was the removal of stockings from the feet. The sexual value of the feet was clear. Rather than the ring, it was the act of putting on the stocking or sock that was the symbol of marriage.

It is a common false belief that with civilization came modesty:

With the return of warriors from the Crusades in the East, the Oriental influences followed. Europe of the Middle Ages accepted many of the comforts of the East. These included the public baths. These baths were tremendously popular in Germany—so popular that the public was quite shameless when it went to the bathhouses.

With the trumpeting of the bathkeeper's horn in the morning, rich and poor, young and old, male and female took to the streets nearly or completely naked, on their way to the baths. Guarinonius complained that "the father runs naked from the house through the streets to the bath with his naked wife and naked children."

Of course, this public nudity had the predictable result: The public steam baths provided a thick fog in which bathers could have their introductions and sexual connections in near-privacy. Because of this "smokescreen," very few citizens were fined for public indecency.

On the island of Bahrain, in the Persian Gulf, a doctor was very careful in examining women. He could not look directly at her private parts. Instead, he had to hold a mirror to her genitals and look at their image in the mirror.

Periods of public modesty and prudery have typically been followed by fetishistic behavior:

The Bourbon reign in France was a time of high morality, even prudery. With the end of this period came a backlash. In 1817 there appeared a group of sexual deviants called Prickers. It started with a lone Frenchman who found delight in pricking the bottoms of women in public. With publicity, the practice soon spread to other parts of Europe, the "prickers" appearing in Hamburg, Munich, Brussels and London. The wide-scale practice of this was last reported in 1821.

It has been suggested that prolonged or extreme restriction of behavior often leads to a backlash of the behavior so severely prohibited:

In Palestine in the Middle Ages, the Bishop of a seaport town complained that after faithfully observing Easter Lent, the women seemed to more than make up for their good behavior at that time. After being good at Christmas, at Easter the women, he said, "shamelessly attract the attention of every man, "as if seized by frenzy they excite the lasciviousness of youths...transforming the holy places into scenes of lewdness." They sang "harlot's songs" and assumed "shameful postures."

Sexual misbehavior could be severely punished in some societies:

In some tribes of Queensland, Australia, a wife was harshly dealt with.

Her husband punished her by applying hot coals to her stomach.

Among the Muria of Bastar, a girl who did not keep herself clean enough or was otherwise neglectful, was punished by being held down and having ashes stuffed into her vagina.

The Kwonga boy of New Guinea who experienced an erection was quick to leave the village. If he was seen with an erection, a woman beat his penis with a stick.

A great number of societies used community pressure to keep their citizens in line:

In 17th-century England, towns punished adulterous women who lived with their husbands, in an indirect way. The man who was considered too weak to keep a cheating wife in tow was the object of the community's scorn. He was punished for being a cuckold by having to "ride skimmington."
   The skimmington was a ladle. Thus, the man was considered living under the force of his wife's ladle. To cure him of this, he was seized by the villagers and mounted on a horse so that he faced the hindquarters. The community made loud music by banging on frying pans and knocking horns and bones together. Then the cuckold was led through the streets, to be beaten by the village women's skimmingtons. This usually motivated corrective action on the part of the husband toward his wife, and also seems to have been very entertaining.

Community morals have frequently been upheld by those who had the most to gain from keeping marriageable women honest:

French people in the 15th century took a very active role in keeping community standards. Many towns had Abbayes de jeunesse, groups of eligible males, from adolescents to older widowers, who monitored the sexual behavior of their villages. They followed the social habits of the husbands and daughters of the town, and made loud and rowdy visits to those girls whose honor was questionable. They also organized other social events for the younger crowd. They channeled violence into pranks and antics, usually directed at those they thought might be living loosely, and kept a watchful eye on the girls and women who would one day become their wives.

It has happened that a culture required honesty in performance of what could be considered a "dishonest" act:

In northern Algeria, the Bashamma did not often indulge in adultery, but when a man and woman decided to have an affair, it was considered proper to pay the fine before committing the adultery.

Manners usually consist of restrictions, and the ancient Chinese had some of the most restrictive manners in the world:

Chinese Confucianism stressed the purity of the relations between the sexes outside the marital bed. Sometimes, the protection of this chastity took on absurd limits. One of the policies to keep the sexes apart was keeping the husband and wife from dressing and undressing together. Etiquette demanded that men and women could not hang their clothes on the same rack.

Often, sexual modesty is absent in a culture, while modesty of a different sort is observed:

The central African Warrua were relatively liberal in their sexual attitudes, compared to other African tribes. However, each man and woman had his or her own fires and food, and ate in complete privacy. They experienced great embarassment and shame if observed in the act of eating.

Manners have not always dealt strictly with modesty; in some cases, being mannerly meant attracting the attentions of others:

In the 1830s, the French woman, in addition to learning other, more subtle manners, tried to perfect the faint. Fainting, in this period, was an appropriate response from a well-mannered lady. There were many reasons for, and consequently many degrees of, fainting. A few of the many different kinds were the blissful faint, the jealous faint and the dramatic faint. Each had its own style and duration.

Victorian America took manners and delicacy to great extremes, as did Victorian Britons:

In the early and mid-19th century, mannered American women sewed lace "pant legs" to be put on pianos. The naked piano leg was thought to be crude and suggestive, and for this reason had to be clothed.

The prudery of England in the 1800s was reflected in their language. "Sweating" was considered crude, and it was only proper to "perspire." This word, in turn, became too distasteful and was replaced with a more demure verb. Instead, those with wet faces, backs and underarms were considered to be "glowing."

It was considered ill-mannered to refer to a woman as pregnant, and soon she was "with child" instead. Again, this language was eventually considered too gross, and thereafter an expectant mother was considered as being "in an interesting condition."

❧

Religious festivals have sometimes required modesty and decorum, while at other times license was thought to be more appropriate to achieve the aims of its participants:

In ancient Athens at Thesmophoria, and in ancient Rome, among the cult of Vesta (patroness of matronly virtue) and at the Feast of Bona Dea, girls and women observed religious occasions by telling dirty jokes, yelling obscenities and carrying phallic symbols. In later times in ancient Rome, the festivity was toned down and dirty jokes were merely whispered into each other's ears.

❧

The rich and titled, because of their power, could often be above modesty:

The servants of the house in the Middle Ages took orders at any and every hour of the day and night. The master and mistress of the house felt no embarassment at giving orders while performing every kind of sex. They ignored the help as they had intercourse, often being served meals as they finished the sexual act.

❧

In the eastern Arab country of Qatar, a woman who was caught naked in her household preserved her modesty not by covering her body, but by covering her head.

❧

Taking the sexual initiative has typically been the male's role. Many cultures, however, allowed the female to sexually approach a male:

The Tanzanian Turu females were extremely well-mannered women. However, this did not prevent them from soliciting the sexual skills of men. Among the Turus, if a woman asked a male for a hoe, or stole a man's sandals, he could be sure to become her lover.

❧

The northern Siberian woman who was in love with a man showed her interest by throwing slugs at him.

❧

The pride that men and women take in their sexuality, and thus their capacity to have children, is common throughout the world. In any society, the ability to have a family is valued. However, some societies are more educated in the science of this matter than others:

In northern Queensland, a Tully River woman could offer no greater insult to a man than to make fun of the fact that he supposedly ejaculated too much semen.

Obscene language has usually been used to shock or offend. But this practice has its flip side:

The New Mexican Mohaves enjoyed giving themselves obscene names, which they became known by. Each sex named themselves with a description of their mate's sexual qualities or characteristics. Usually, they were very unflattering. The men called themselves "Charcoal Vagina," "25-Cent Vagina," "Copulates Incessantly," "Vagina Full With Fleas" or some such insult. In retaliation the women, as a reflection on their husbands, called themselves, among other things, "Charcoal Testicles," "Pound His Penis" or "Rotten Rectum."

In the country of Laos, women were not allowed to go barefoot or wear sandals. The exposure of female toes was considered obscene. A husband punished his wife's bad behavior by taking away her shoes—forcing her to stay in her hut until he gave her shoes back.

The church, for a very long time, was the primary legislator of morals:

In the late 16th century, Thomas Sanchez advised that the only natural position for sex was with the woman on her back and the man on top. The female dominant position was strictly forbidden, and to prove its sinfulness, a theologian claimed that because some women insisted on the reversal of positions, "God had sent the Flood to destroy mankind."

In New Mexico, among some tribes, a man could not approach his wife for sex for a week after she had finished her period. He could not even touch her. After a week, she took a bath, and the couple was finally allowed to make love. If it was ever found out that he had violated this custom, he was put to death.

In a large number of cultures, there have been taboos regarding sex with a pregnant woman:

The New Guinean Arapesh people forbade sexual activity between man and wife once the woman's breasts became large and tender—the indications of pregnancy. It was claimed that the baby should not be "awakened" through sexual intercourse between father and mother. This restriction was taken further if the man had more than one wife. If one wife became pregnant, the father could have no intercourse with any of his wives.

❧

Among the Chinese of the Middle Ages, it was common to urinate standing up, whereas in later times they performed this function squatting. Very wealthy or titled men often carried a cane, not only for the purposes of walking, but also for the purpose of urinating with dignity. The cane was wide enough to allow the gentleman to insert his penis. He urinated through the cane, the urine flowing through the cane and onto the ground much less conspicuously than the standard method.

❧

There has occurred extreme liberalism in matters of sexuality and privacy:

The ancient Lacedaemonians kept track of the fitness of their army by public inspections. They watched for signs of physical slackness by insisting that the army parade once a week in the nude.

❧

In France in the 18th century, members of the opposite sex refused to be embarrassed by a companion's call to the toilet. They merely followed their friends into the water closet and kept talking while their companions sat and relieved themselves.

❧

It was not uncommon for women in 17th-century Spain to expose their breasts in public. This was not considered obscene or ill-mannered. However, her feet were never to be exposed in public; they were to be seen by nobody except her husband.

❧

Rather than cover their pubic hair, Bismarck Archipelago women took advantage of the unusually large amount of hair on their pubis, and used it as a kind of cloth with which they wiped their hands.

❧

While very modest in public, the Samoans had a very open sexual atmosphere at home. While they did not so much as touch hands in public or even walk side by side, a couple could celebrate their wedding night with a vigorous bout of intercourse in a hut with 10 other people present.

Restriction of pleasure has often been viewed as a sign of respect for the dead:

Confucianist Chinese mourning the loss of a parent abstained from sex for three years after the unhappy occasion. Should a wife have showed signs of pregnancy before the expiry date, friends and relatives shunned the couple.

Other Confucians were even more demanding concerning the showing of respect to ancestors. They denied themselves sex on the anniversaries of their parents' and grandparents' deaths. They also refrained from taking their sexual pleasure on the birthdays of their wives and concubines, out of respect for the pain their mothers endured during childbirth.

Some customs may survive long after the reason for the practice has been forgotten:

An ancient English custom continued into the 19th century in the town of Coventry. One particular day each year, a girl was chosen from a number of willing candidates to ride down the main street nude, as Lady Godiva did in 1057. After her ride, she was escorted to dinner by the mayor of Coventry, and they dined together—she still stark naked.

A strange custom occurred up until the 19th century in Hertfordshire, England. Every seven years, on October 10, young men gathered and chose a leader. They took an oath of loyalty to their head man and set out on their wanderings. They traveled all day until late that night.

The young men treated all whom they met to a bit of exercise. Boy or girl, they picked up the "victim" and swung them about. The young men, of course, favored swinging the skirted women, exposing the girls' charms. The more virtuous girls were, for this reason, confined indoors. The looser women allowed the exercise and accompanied the young men on the rest of their tour.

Political, military and physical power have always been equated with sexual power:

In ancient Iraq, the most powerful and respected of the Caliphs took the title Resheed, which meant "guided on the right path"—into a woman's vagina. The ancient Persians had a similar designation for men of reputation—Ali, or Futteh Khan ("Conqueror of Virgins; Opener of Vaginae").

Medieval knights acted according to a code of chivalry, but this code did provide for satisfying his sexual appetite. Should a knight have come across a woman, and she was alone, he acted with the utmost decency and politeness. If he came across a woman in the company of another knight, however, he could challenge the knight. If he succeeded in killing the enemy knight, the woman was his prize—to treat in any way he wished. She had no say in the manner in which he treated her, regardless if she found him repulsive and wished to refuse his advances. The victorious knight could even prostitute her.

According to the Confucianists, the Chinese husband and wife could not keep their clothes in the same place until both partners had reached the age of 70. It was forbidden for a husband and his wife to directly hand each other anything. Except during funeral or sacrificial ceremonies, the woman offered the male objects by presenting them on a tray. It was also in this way that she received items from him.

A reduction in the social and moral standards has often resulted in the justification of otherwise deviant behavior, with a decidedly sexual tone:

During the year of the Black Death in Germany, in 1349, a group of Hungarian women entered into that country and introduced a form of religious penance. These women tore their clothes off in public, sang songs and whipped and beat themsevles with scourges and rods. They were known as the Flagellants, and soon thousands of men and women across Europe, 800,000 in France alone, were joining in nude processions through the streets, appealing to God to stop the suffering, and mortifying their flesh.

A somewhat common occurrence between cultures is the use of what is considered sin to purify oneself:

Shortly after the Black Death started sweeping through Europe, it was believed that committing incest on the church altar was the only prescription against infection with the Plague virus.

In 16th-century Brazil, the white colonists believed that a man suffering from venereal disease could be cured by sleeping with a black virgin.

Modesty has, at times, reached extremes:

In the time of the Chinese Ming dynasty (1368–1644), doctors were not allowed to see female patients nude. Instead, the patient stood behind a curtain and offered her hand to the doctor. The physician made his diagnosis by taking the woman's pulse. The closest that doctors came to seeing the locale of women's ailments was through a carved ivory model of the female figure, which the doctor carried with him. The husband or a female relative of the woman, not she herself, pointed to the area of complaint on the doll.

❍⚮

It was only in the late 19th century that doctors were allowed into Arab harems. Even then, the doctors had extremely restricted access to the women. When examining a sultana, a very large and strong eunuch stood by. The girl stood behind a black curtain. The doctor diagnosed her illness by examining her tongue, which she stuck through a hole in the curtain.

❍⚮

Some customs emphasize the inferiority of a wife to her husband; others emphasize the power of the husband in his capacity as hunter or warrior over his wife:

The 17th-century Spanish king observed a ritual that underscored his wife's status not so much as queen, but as a subject. He was always required to enter the queen's bedchamber ready for the amorous battle, wearing domestic slippers and a black cape over his shoulder. He also had a shield on one arm, a sword in the other, an extinguished lantern, and a bottle that he would use as a chamberpot. It was in this costume and with these accessories that he always entered his queen's chambers, unescorted.

❍⚮

The Arab sultan was an all-powerful man, and often, in his position, he had to be ruthless. However, this very powerful, ruthless man, before picking his bed partner from among his many women, had to go to his mother and show his humility and submission to her.

❍⚮

The Middle Eastern harem owner followed a certain protocol that seems to have emphasized his indifference in choosing his bedmate. The girl chosen, in turn, showed the utmost respect in manners for her master:

The Persian harem owner determined his sexual partner for the night in a very democratic way. It was called Tremmehel-mehre—"the tossing of the handkerchief." He gathered his wives together in a room and produced a handkerchief. The woman who accompanied her master to bed was the one on whose shoulder his tossed handkerchief fell.

Whenever a girl of the harem was called on to lay with her master for a night of pleasure, she was very careful to observe his authority and show her subservience, even in the conjugal bed. Her approach to him was a humble crawl.

The harem master was already in bed when she was ushered in. A

34

sultan's bedmate was usually allowed to claim any money that he had in his clothing, and she usually went through his pockets before going to bed with the sultan.

To show her respect, instead of climbing into bed beside him, she pulled up the sheet at the end of the bed and crawled up to the head of the bed under the covers.

Urine was considered by many African tribes as "holy water," and essential in safeguarding those who needed to be blessed:

The Bakitara king of central Africa had a female chamberlain who was responsible for urinating on his feet in the morning so that he could successfully start the day.

Sex has been primarily a private matter. But this has not precluded enjoying it outside of the house:

The ancient Chinese desired to have "heaven as a witness" to copulation, and thus outdoor sexual activity was very popular. The very rich built beautiful gardens with high walls for this very purpose.

Usually a couple will live together to strengthen the union and facilitate sexual activity. This is not always the case:

Among the American Zuni Indians, the husband was not allowed to enter his wife's house, even for a visit. Their sexual attachment took place at night on the porch.

Some cultures have restricted the number of days when one could have sex:

In ancient China, as with Western civilizations, there were certain days when sex was not allowable. According to the Yellow Calendar, after tallying the dates unsuitable for sex, lovers had about 100 days' worth of lovemaking per year.

Though it is hard to imagine love and courtship without the kiss, it has been so. The kiss has not always been a sign of affection, nor has it always been a part of love or manners:

When western travelers first explored China, the Chinese were quite horrified at the insulting habit of kissing. The French Indo-Chinese mothers disciplined their misbehaving children by threatening to give them a "European kiss."

The Tahitian kiss was the Ho'i—lovers rubbing and sniffing their noses. The European kiss on the mouth was considered a perversion. In one instance observed, a woman complained that her husband was so disgustingly drunk, he'd tried to "European kiss" her.

There are many degress of friendship and respect displayed when greeting another person:

The central Australian Walibri men, when visiting each other's villages, showed the sign of friendship by shaking each other's penises.

There are varying degrees of intimacy associated with kissing:

A form of kissing more commom than the lip-to-lip kiss was the "smell kiss." It was considered mannerly for boys to raise their loincloths to women, who "smell kissed" his penis.

At times, politeness has been sacrificed in the interests of sexual morality:

At one time, clerics could not speak directly to women. After the church became aware of the sexual excesses of its clergy, in the 11th century Pope Leo IX and Peter Damiani provided that holy men were not allowed to even talk to women. The penalty for disobeying this order was 100 to 200 lashes.

The Banyai son-in-law was a virtual slave to his new mother-in-law. He was obligated to provide firewood for her for the rest of his life. He had to approach her on his knees, because should his feet point toward her, she would be insulted.

As was the custom, the Californian Modoc son-in-law did his best to avoid meeting his mother-in-law. Should he unavoidably meet her, however, he was obligated to kill her.

The polite New Englander played host by offering his guests his bed to "bundle" in:

Bundling was the act of a man and a woman going to bed fully clothed. Bundling occured in New England as an act of hospitality of the colonial people toward travelers who, very often, had no hotel to stop in at. As well, there were not many diversions in the evening for the frontier settler, so lovers tended to retire early. This also saved on firewood. Often there was a shortage of firewood, so when the fire went out, they found the only warmth in bed.

It was considered very good manners for a husband to give up his place in bed to a person stopping at his house. He offered his place in the bed beside his wife, whether the guest was female or male.

~

There have been many different degrees of hospitality and mannerliness:

The wife in an ancient Chinese household was considered almost a nonentity. She kept herself anonymous, and her husband paid little or no attention to her. In fact, it was considered a great insult for a guest to ask the husband about his wife.

In central Africa there lived the Banyankole tribe. While visiting friends, husbands exchanged wives for the length of their stay.

The North American Missouri Indians felt the obligation to provide guests with sexual companionship, just as many other tribes allowed visitors to share their wives. However, the Missouris were less generous. The guest did not get to know the host's wife sexually; instead, he was provided with a slave for this purpose.

The Iroquois Indian males could give their wives over, for a time, to anyone they so desired, as a gesture of friendship. This was a very common practice; however, they considered sexual relations with a woman not given as a gift as the most outrageous insult.

Sioux Indian males considered it the grossest insult if the offer of their wife to a guest or a friend was turned down. However, should the man so treated attempt a second sexual interview with the wife, without having been offered her, he would be killed.

~

While hosts could be very generous, the guest might sometimes be called on to show his brotherhood in a difficult way:

The Russian Koryak people observed a custom of friendship. Before welcoming a stranger in, the host's wife emptied her bladder of urine into a jar in his presence. The stranger was then offered the contents of her toilet. As a sign of friendship, the visitor took the jar and rinsed his mouth with her urine.

~

The status of women could be threatened if they were not married in the proper way, by show of their worth. Breach of social custom could be a severe matter:

37

In southern Australia lived the Narrinyeri. A woman who was not bought with another woman by her husband-to-be was disgraced. Should the young stag not have had a sister to trade for his wife, he bought the right to one of his cousins.

A Yakut woman was humiliated if she was not married by purchase. When notified of the European custom of marriage, the natives considered the European women quite shameless. In the event that a man would or could not buy her, she offered him a dowry as an incentive to buy her.

The Cammorista woman of Italy measured the love her husband had for her by the extent to which her husband was willing to beat her. The more consistent the beatings, the greater his love, and the man who refused to demonstrate this was considered an idiot.

⚮

The faithfulness of widows and widowers has been variable, according to the culture:

An East Indian woman married in the ceremonial style was very inhibited if she was widowed. A widow who spoke to or was familiar with a man within four years of her husband's death was charged with adultery.

The South American Siriono were careful to abstain from sex as a sign of respect when a husband or wife died. This sign of respect for the dead spouse lasted all of two or three days.

The East Indian widow so desired to remain faithful to her husband that she often argued with his other wives over who would be allowed to be killed on his gravesite. The loyal wife also fought his other wives for the honor of being with him on the Suttee, or funeral pyre, which cremated him.

⚮

African tribes showed respect for their tribe members in special ways:

Among the Whydah, upon the death of a villager, the rest of the village mourned for one year. During this time, all the tribe refrained from sex.

If there had been bloodshed in the death of a Kikamba tribeswoman, a stranger was enlisted to make love to and sleep with the corpse. In the morning, he found a cow in front of the hut—his to keep.

⚮

In Baluchistan, in India, a husband who suspected a stranger of having sex with his wife in public was the model of discretion. The husband said nothing, but quietly left her alone. Should he have later arrived at

38

his house to see shoes sitting outside the door, he made loud noises to allow the couple time to separate and the man to leave.

❦

In most primitive cultures, nudity has been natural. There have been different degrees of modesty, though:

Among some tribes in Africa, it was common that women went topless and men had minimal coverings for their genitals. However, it was considered obscene for a man or woman to be sitting down with the bottoms of the feet exposed.

Among the Brazilian Urubu tribe, nudity was common, and naked citizens walked around unashamed. The male was required to have his foreskin tied up over the head of his penis with a string, concealing the head of the penis. To be seen without his "wrapped prepuce" was a humiliation. The men, in an effort to hide the head, even urinated in a squatting position, whereas the females of the tribe urinated standing up.

❦

It has been a feature of well-mannered societies that individuals conduct their sexual contacts in private. At least one society, however, put the onus on the public to provide privacy:

The Mangaians of the South Pacific showed great freedom. Couples freely made love in the most public of places. Huts housed up to 15 people in the same room, but this did not prevent anyone from having sex in the hut for all to see. Instead of the lovers seeking privacy to have sex, the members of the family and tribe took care to look away. The fathers of unmarried daughters, who usually had sex with several different boyfriends, paid no attention to the sexplay.

❦

At times, public nudity has been perfectly acceptable:

The Arabs of the Middle Ages were modest in terms of dress and manner. However, this extreme restriction of dress could be cast aside as a true sign of despair on the part of an upset man or woman. The Arab messenger showed his compassion to the receiver of bad news by tearing his clothing. A mother at wit's end in convincing her child of something or other, frequently abandoned her clothes as a sign of her reckless despair at their behavior. Women in mourning tore their clothes and threw away their veils, and also exposed their breasts.

The people of France in the Middle Ages continued a pagan practice of forming public processions. These processions marched through the streets, appealing to the gods for a change in political, military or economic fortunes. At first the people merely walked barefoot, but

39

with the passage of time they removed more and more garments to show the gods their humility. By 1224, all clothes were removed for these marches. For at least 100 years, these processions were frequent in Paris, though it was usually only men, not women, who stripped down.

♀

Sex has been a large feature of war in every culture, in every age, whether it be to capture women or show an army's male superiority:

In 326 B.C. Alexander the Great (356–323 B.C.), King of Macedonia, was victorious over the Persians and Indians at the Hydaspes River. To celebrate the victory, 30,000 captive women and Macedonians had intercourse on a Kashmir mountainside.

Sesostris, the Egyptian king around 3700 B.C., erected columns as monuments to his conquering armies. After defeating an especially brave and proud army, he erected columns showing the heroic struggle and eventual victory of his forces.

When he encountered little oppostion to his invasions, and weak resistance was offered, he took another approach. The columns he erected in the localities where cowardice was shown belittled the men of that area. The sculptured columns showed the female genitals, accusing the losers of having fought like women.

An Anglo-Egyptian army fought in Africa in the late 19th century. This army was led by Pasha Hicks. With the slaughter of Hicks' army by the Mahdi in Kordofan Province, the leader of the victorious army threw the penises of 10,000 of Hicks' men into a well near El-Obeyd. The women of the city of El-Obeyd wore the testicles of the defeated men on their clothing, as if they were tassels.

During World War II, the German army planted "castration mines." A soldier stepping on the booby trap triggered the mine to explode. The explosion catapulted the mine to about the area of the soldier's groin, then exploded again, which, at the very least, castrated the unfortunate soldier.

In the fighting between the northern Balkan people of Montenegro and those of Albania, it was common for the Albanian females to play an active role in the clashes. These women stood in the front lines, and in a show of magical incantation, cast a spell which they thought would ensure victory. They did this by lifting their skirts and exposing their vaginas to the enemy.

The Afridi woman followed her countrymen into battle and castrated all who fell in front of her. She also played an active role in torturing prisoners: While a stick braced the prisoners' mouths open, this "she wolf" urinated into their mouths, and these unfortunate wounded men drowned in her urine.

In some cultures, there have existed severe nudity taboos, creating great shame among citizens:

In old Ireland, people were extremely modest; even bare feet could embarrass both the barefooted and the observer. In some Irish villages, the citizens followed the habit of modestly changing their clothes underneath the bedcovers.

Dutch New Guinea pygmy males wore nothing but a foot-long wooden gourd, which they placed around their penises.

New Hebrides men were very modest concerning their penises. This was not because of any sexual custom. Rather, the sight of a penis had magical powers. For this reason, the otherwise naked male wrapped his member in several yards of cloth, and the resulting covering could be as big as two feet long.

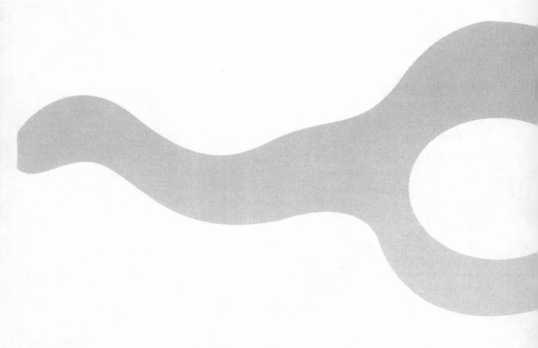

SEX AND RELIGION

Regulation of sexual relations has been a concern for churches even when lascivious conduct was not likely:

In old Ireland, the congregation was distinctly divided four ways at church. Adult males and females sat apart in their own sections of the church. Boys and girls also formed their own separate groups. The four groups could not mix until they left the church, each group leaving separately.

Sex has been associated with religious faith and good fortune, because it implied fertility and thus prosperity:

Beginning in the time of the Han dynasty, the Chinese collected "spring coins." These rectangular coins featured a lucky saying on one side and a representation of a god and goddess making love on the other.

There have been extremely sex-negative religious groups:

There were certain religious sects that taught disgust for the reproductive act. This usually included various forms of self-denial, including castration. Such believers were the Albigensians, Bulgars and Cathars. The Cathars had such a repulsion of sex that they were vegetarians. They would not eat meat, cheese, milk or eggs, because these were products of animals, which had sex.

In ancient Rome, a religious sect called the Valesians believed that castration was the only way to be pure. For this reason, they castrated themselves—and others, who they tried to save from sin.

The Scopts, a radical religious cult formed in the 18th century, were an offshoot of England's Dissenters. The majority of Scopts settled in Russia, where they practiced deprivation and flagellation. Subsequently, the main feature of their baptismal ceremony was castration. They believed that Christ was castrated and preached castration, as a reaction to the misfortune that befell Adam and Eve in the Garden of Eden.

In ancient history, the phallus was an important part of religious worship and symbolism:

Phallic worship was popular in ancient Greece. The Greek historian Herodotus (485–425 B.C.) noted that women carried representations of the male part which were as large as the women carrying them.

In some parts of France until the early 1800s, citizens celebrated Easter with pinnes. *Pinne* was a dirty word meaning "penis." Women baked little loaves of bread shaped like penises, and women and children carried them on palm branches during processions. They then saved the pinnes for the rest of the year as good-luck charms.

Men called Kuzzibash, Moslem mystics whose history goes back at least to the 13th century, frequently painted their penises red, green or yellow.

The Greek fertility god Dionysus was worshiped by the appearance of phalluses, sexually explicit skits and drunken orgies. Originally he was not a god in human form but was represented as a huge, erect penis.

In Madagascar in the 17th century, a strange ceremony was observed. The holy man cut off a boy's foreskin with his sharpened fingernails. After it was dipped in egg yolk, the boy's godfather swallowed the foreskin.

The phallic symbol was also used to ensure fertility:

As sons were considered a source of wealth among the Hindus, male offspring were always preferred. Hindu women who became pregnant and desired a male could visit a shrine, impale themselves on a magical lingham, or penis, and be assured that they would deliver a son.

Holy men have commonly been enlisted to change the sexual fortunes of women:

In ancient Rome, to honor the wife of Faustulus, who raised Romulus and Remus, the founders of Rome, the Lupercalia was held every

February 15. Young men raced through the streets naked, hitting any woman they could find in range, with a thong. Women made themselves available for this occasion, believing that they would become more fertile after having taken blows from these nude runners.

The Egyptian maslub, or saint, was believed to have the power to render women fertile merely by their kneeling in front of him. The maslub traveled completely naked, which accommodated his habit of initiating sexual intercourse with any woman he so desired, on the spot. Her envious friends celebrated her good fortune by dancing and singing during the spectacle and offering their congratulations.

The French in the Middle Ages were told by their clergy that sex with a priest would bless a woman. While other women were considered adulteresses, the priests' mistresses were held in high esteem.

Nor have only women received the attentions of the privileged holy man:

Baghdad was home to a Barmecide cult between A.D. 700 and 800. Barmecides were also found in Afghanistan. The mystic of this cult was called a Derweesh, Soofee or Mejzood. Unlike most people in those parts, the mystic, unlike ordinary people, was allowed to urinate in the middle of the road instead of at the roadside.

It was the mystic's privilege to enlist any boy or man to offer his anus to the mystic's passions. When meeting the priest, the respectful traveler kissed him, in sequence, on the mouth, navel, penis, scrotum and buttocks.

In Byblos, Syria, the ancient Syrians celebrated the death of Adonis. At this festival, the women shaved off their hair and beat their breasts as a sign of distress. If the women didn't want to shave their hair off, they had to prostitute themselves for a day and give the money to the Temple of Aphrodite.

Initiation ceremonies for priests of some religions could be very demanding:

In ancient Rome, around 191 B.C., a cult called the Galli worshiped the goddess Cybele. They held four-day festivals in the spring in which members were initiated by slashing their own arms and backs. On the third day of celebrations, the Day of Blood, a young Galli man took a sword into his hands and castrated himself.

Holding his severed genitals in hand, he ran as fast as he could through the streets for as long as he could. When exhausted, he flung his genitals through the nearest window, whereupon he received women's clothes and accessories.

The ancient Roman practice of fertility worship and deflowering a new bride on a "holy phallus" managed to survive several centuries:

A church in Orange, France, wrecked during the French Revolution, revealed in its basement a relic from the past. It was a phallic object used to pray for the penis' potence and health. It was long and wooden and covered with leather. It may have been inserted into the virgin bride (the reason for the leather covering), in much the same way the Roman bride was deflowered.

The church has served primarily as a place of worship, but in some cases it had an even more practical aspect:

The Archbishop of Canterbury, Odo, built a passageway in Ripon Cathedral's crypt. This specially built passageway was of such dimensions, Odo claimed, that only a virgin could pass through.

The church has not always been a place of piety and dignity:

The officials of Italian churches during the Renaissance welcomed high-class prostitutes, called courtesans, into the church. These women were welcomed because their presence advertised the churches they attended. These women, some of the most beautiful and well-dressed in Italy, were in fact drawing cards for the churches. Many men attended church to witness the courtesans' beauty or to find one for their pleasure; women went to check out the latest fashions.

Churches of the Middle Ages did not contain just images of Jesus, the Virgin Mary or the saints. Alongside more pious paintings and sculptures were those showing the bawdier side of the clergy. Churches in England, France, Holland and the Mediterranean all featured comic representations of the church hierarchy. The craftsmen who made these images were lay brothers and monks who often enjoyed poking fun at their superiors. The subjects of these artworks were priests exposing their buttocks and private parts, making faces and chasing women. They also characterized the priests as pigs, monkeys and rats. Nuns, bishops and abbots were all shown carousing in various ways.

A church near Geneva featured a fresco depicting sodomites practicing their preference. A Vezelay church showed a female saint exposing herself. A Strasbourg church pulpit had a carving of a monk and a nun, the monk's hand snaked up her habit and thrust between the nun's legs.

The church administration, holding no illusions about priests or the congregation's views of church officers and clerics, let these needlings go without much complaint.

Old Irish churches often featured a good-luck charm carved into the keystone of the arch over the doorway. This charm protected all who passed under it from the evil eye. The charm above the church door: a carved stone image of a squatting woman exposing her genitals.

For much of the church's existence, it has had to contend with rival phallus worship. In some cases, the church had to share the congregation's attentions along with pagan rites:

From the 16th century in Languedoc, Lyonnaise and Provence in southern France, and St. Tens in Antwerp, St. Foutin was represented by a huge wooden phallus. Women scraped the phallus and boiled the shavings in water as a remedy for sterility. Wax phalluses were hung from the ceilings of churches—swaying in the drafts. There is evidence that young girls gave their virginity to the artificial phallus of St. Foutin.

In Isernia, in the kingdom of Naples, Italy, young girls and infertile women, starting every September 27, worshipped St. Cosmo, St. Foutin and St. Damiano. This three-day festival of phallic worship was part of the church ceremony held in a church dedicated to Cosmo and Damiano. The female worshipers stayed nights in the church, bringing with them wax replicas of the erect penis. They kissed the wax penises and handed them to the priests, saying, "Blessed St. Cosmo, that's how I want it to be," or "Blessed St. Cosmo, let it be like this." As a result of their overnight stays in the church, with the blessings of the priests, many girls and women, nine months later, showed the obvious signs of fertility.

Men who wanted to make their own members vigorous said a prayer to St. Cosmo and St. Damiano, and exposed their private parts at the altar. The priest sprinkled it with holy oil. The sale and distribution of oil of St. Cosmo and Damiano was so popular that 1,400 flasks of it were recorded used in 1780.

Pagan rites coexisted and sometimes dominated Christian holidays:

In the time of Pope Leo X, during the time of Lent, "there is in Rome a...Carne-vale which endureth the space of three or four days; all which time the Pope keepeth himself out of Rome." Costume and cross-dressing was a feature of this carnival: "The gentlemen will attyre themselves...some like women, others like Turkes." Of course, all this happened where the sexual entertainment was located: "And all this is done where the courtizanes be to show them delight and pastime." And, of course, this social and sexual pandemonium had to have its element of violence: "If anyone bear a secret malice to another, he may kill him, and nobody will lay hands on him."

Pagan phallic rituals and worship for a very long time coexisted with Christianity:

From the beginning of Christianity, phallic worship rivaled it for the faith of the followers. In times of disaster, it was often considered an option after the Christian methods of appealing for God's mercy had failed. Such an incident occurred in 1268. A widespread pestilence infested the Lothian district of Scotland, killing the cattle. Christian ceremonies and appeals did not seem to cure the disaster.

The frustrated clergymen finally instructed the Lothians to build a fire and erect a statue of a phallus to save the cattle. The cattle were also sprinkled with holy water in which dogs' testicles had been soaked.

When a similar disaster struck the county of Fife in Scotland, a priest, finding no change in fortune with Christian prayer, turned to phallic worship. A huge phallus was raised up. The priest chanted and sang obscene phrases. The young girls of the area took his example and did the same while they danced naked around the symbol of Priapus.

In regulating sexual behavior, religion has often policed behavior in other, far-reaching areas of life:

The church of the Middle Ages considered the theater sinful, because in ancient Rome, the themes were explicit, and there was frequently on-stage nudity. For this reason, the church considered wearing costume or disguise a sin. This imitation, called mumming, could not be practiced by Christians, and thus no Christian could be an actor or even marry one. Thus, because of the sexual nature of ancient Roman theater, persons centuries later were excommunicated, and frequently executed, for wearing costume.

The Catholic Church released its manifesto on the hunting and persecution of witches, *Malleus Maleficarum* ("Hammer of the Female Witches"). This work was challenged by Reginald Scot's text, in 1487, called *The Discoverie of Witchcraft*. In it, Scot opposed the methods of the holy exorcists, who, in the name of driving the evil from the witch's body, considered it necessary to take suspected witches to the altar and have sex with them.

Religious rituals have involved almost every type of deviant sexual behavior known in the name of worship:

In northern Italy and southern France in the 12th and 13th centuries, there lived a religious sect called Catharistic Manicheans. The males of these believers used to spread their sperm on slices of bread and eat the product in celebration of the Last Supper.

In 1233, Pope Gregory IX denounced the practice of the Osculum Infame among religious heretics. The French Albigensians reportedly held their religious ceremonies in caves, and the Osculum Infame, or "Obscene Kiss," was one of the rituals performed. The procedure involved the members of the congregation kissing the buttocks or anus of an animal. In some sects, the "Bishop" had his congregation kiss his bared buttocks and inserted a silver spoon into his anus.

Egyptian religious ceremonies often involved bestiality. Women frequently had sex with goats, which represented the Sacred Goat of Mendas.

In Athens, Greece, each year a young woman was selected to represent Queen Archon. The queen had married Dionysis. Dionysis was represented by a bull, so in the ceremony the girl was "married" to the bull. Afterward the girl had sex with the bull in the cattle stall.

Morality has not always been enough to satisfy religious institutions:

During the middle of the 13th century, Pope Innocent III commanded the execution of the Albigense people by papal troops. The Albigensians were very moral people. Even their enemies admitted this, but nonetheless their beliefs ran counter to the church's beliefs, so they were exterminated.

The Brethren of the Free Spirit did not conform to the church, either. These German people were very moral, mannered people as well. Unfortunately, they were also nudists. They met the same fate as the Albigensians—exterminated by the papal army.

A natural result of public worship was the presence of orgies. There have been innumerable variations on this ritual:

A curious religious sect, believed to be Cathars, lived near Soissons, France, in the 12th century. These worshipers did not have a temple and met in secret. Candles were lit and women bared their buttocks to men who stood behind them. The candles were put out, and the room was consumed in darkness. All together, they yelled "Chaos!" grabbed a member of the opposite sex and had intercourse.

In the 11th century, a religious sect called the Patrini emerged in Milan, Italy. Their religious ceremony was closed and very private. At sundown they closed the doors and windows of their temples. All were quiet. A large black cat on a rope came down from the ceiling. The lights were extinguished and each member in turn took the cat. Some kissed its feet, others kissed under its tail, still others kissed its genitals. After these devotions, they picked a member of the opposite sex closest to them, and orgied.

Women who produced children took them to the private "temple." The congregation encircled a well-fed fire. The infant was tossed across the fire from person to person. Once it was slow-broiled to death, it was thrown into the fire. The ashes of the dead infant were the main ingredient of a sacramental bread, which was eaten by the congregation.

The 16th-century Indian religious sect, Caitanya, was well known for having group sex along with the religious ceremonies. The ceremonies were performed, then parishioners gave themselves up to orgies.

Another Indian religious group from the Sakti sect, the Kauchiluas, practiced "religious" sexual intercourse. The women and girls each placed an article in a chest. Upon finishing the spiritual part of the ceremony, the males of the congregation lined up to pick an article out of the chest. It was in this way that men and women paired off with each other for sex. This was presided over by a priest and often included incestuous pairings.

In many religions, sexual anger was directed toward the opposite sex, or even sex in general:

Afghanistan had a radical religious sect call Chiraugh-Kushnee. It also had chapters in India and Persia. These men called themselves the Lamp Extinguishers because they wished to extinguish the "light of procreation." They hated women and feared the overpopulation of the world. They prevented any sexual attraction to women by vigorously and continually masturbating. In this way their organs were perpetually tired and extremely sensitive, so that penetration of a woman could not be accomplished.

In India there lived a religious group of women called She-Wolves and Pye-Dogs. These women traveled in bands and spent their time ambushing men and painfully sacrificing them to the Dark Mother of Destruction. Victims were tortured, raped, castrated and decapitated. Often, the Singhisstreeyun, or "Tiger Woman," performed an operation that proceeded from pleasure to agony. She masturbated the helpless victim slowly and constantly, until he was driven senseless.

It has been common for worship to take place outside churches and temples, and celebrations to become citywide events:

St. Agatha was martyred by her death at the hands of Emperor Decius in A.D. 251, and the circumstances of her death led to strange processions in celebration of her. She was tortured by Decius' men, and his governor, aggravated at her dignity through all the cruelty, ordered her breasts abused and then cut them off.

Every spring and autumn, residents of southern Italy celebrated St. Agatha's Festival by ringing the bells, parading through the streets with relics and carrying gigantic breasts.

In ancient Greece, citizens had a nine-day celebration in autumn celebrating the Eleusinian Mysteries. The first five days were concerned with pilgrimages to the sea to purify themselves. This stripping of clothes and bathing was frequently done with something less than the purest of motives. Afterward, the travelers journeyed from Athens to Eleusis. Once they reached Eleusis, they vigorously celebrated. Part of these celebrations included incestuous sex.

The Hindus celebrated spring festivals called Hoolee and fall festivals called Dewalee. The well-mannered, serious Hindu was transformed into a wild, sex-crazy lunatic. Great crowds of Hindus ran about the streets, yelling, banging on drums and singing obscene songs. Strapped to the men's waists were three-foot-long wooden phalluses. They thrust these penises forward with their hips, imitating the sex act.

Some East Indian religious festivals celebrated the fertility of women. In these celebrations, a red dye called Gulual was squirted and smeared on people and buildings. There was also loud chanting and banging on drums to celebrate the female menstrual habit.

Along with the quiet, pious observance of holy days, history has had its fair share of bawdy holidays:

The French during the Renaissance had a custom that permitted the male to view the nude female. During the Feast of the Holy Innocents, males contrived to surprise females in the act of dressing or undressing and slapped them on the buttocks. This was called "innocenting" and was frequently used as an excuse to satisfy the male curiosity as to a certain female's personal charms.

To release sexual tensions, days were put aside when absurdity and indulgence were the rule:

For about 10 centuries, starting in the seventh century A.D., the French celebrated a festival called the Feast of Fools. In it, concealed desires, especially those of the holy men, were released. A donkey was led into the church. A special satirical hymn was created for the occasion, and at the end of every verse, the singers brayed like asses. People drank wine and later expelled it from either their stomachs or their bladders, in public. They swore and made obscene gestures. Women were willing subjects in sexual play. The congregation repeated the Mass backward and, instead of burning incense, cooked sausages and puddings. The clergy dressed in costumes or women's clothes. At the altar they played dice, ate and sang off-color songs while Mass was being held.

Often, the congregation orgied. Later, a church order obligated them to go outside the church before indulging in sex. The priests rode about town in dung carts, singing obscene songs and hitting the townspeople with lumps of manure.

☼

More moral churchmen refused to indulge in such festivities:

Priests who refused to engage in the Feast of Fools were praised by their superiors, but not necessarily by the congregation. In 1498, some citizens of Tournai, in present-day Belgium, punished their holy men for refusing to practice the same sort of fun they were having. They were taken in hand, stripped half-naked, and led to a tavern, where they were locked up for several days—no doubt to force them to drink liquor to stay alive.

☼

At times the promise of Heaven could be too remote for those faced with immediate death:

During the Middle Ages, the European syphilis epidemic killed one-third of all Europeans. Doctors had no cure for the disease and sufferers died a slow and painful death. Desperate to get all the pleasure out of their lives that they could, the population indulged in sex even more.

Nuns became afraid that they might die unfulfilled, so they left the convents to orgy with the rest of the population. Unfortunately, for the most part it only exposed them to more infection and the death they were so afraid of.

☼

The issue of marriage amongst the clergy was one that lasted a long time and was dealt with in many different ways:

In the 11th century, Pope Leo IX and Peter Damiani began the moral "cleaning up" of the clergy. Much of their energies were concerned with removing sex from the holy man's life. This included separating him from his sexual past. To do this, the church took away all the children the clerical men had fathered with concubines, and made them slaves of the church.

In the 13th century, Pope Alexander III directed the Bishop of Exeter to weed out those subdeacons who needed to be married and those who were not fit to be so. The pope declared that those holy men of bad character and loose morals would be a threat to the females of his parish and so should keep their wives. Those priests who were of good and regular habits would be safe from the congregation as unmarried men. Thus, these men should have their wives taken away from them.

The church under Pope Urban II was set against marriage of the clergy. The church enacted a strict policy in eliminating clerical sexual practices, which, while it may have hurt the priests, had an even worse impact on their wives. Under a papal order, priests' wives were given away to noblemen—as slaves—or taken by the bishops as slaves to the church.

Religious intolerance has plagued lovers since the beginning of religious belief. Some tender lovers were the victims of religious discrimination and suffered humiliation because of their love for someone with the "wrong" faith:

In 14th-century England, the medieval Christian Church regarded intercourse between Christians and Jews as a horrible sin. It was the law that "those who are connected to Jews or Jewesses or are guilty of bestiality or sodomy shall be buried alive in the ground."

Religious persecution toward some Jews was at least temporarily solved by a simple but painful operation:

Jews in the time of the Holy Roman Empire were constantly harassed because of their faith. They were persecuted mercilessly for their beliefs, and part of this persecution took the form of extremely high taxes. All known Jews were required to be examined regularly to confirm their Jewishness. Very often, the man suspected of being a Jew was forced to take his clothes off in public. Then his penis was publicly examined, because circumcision was proof of his Jewishness.

Church policy has at times seemed extremely severe toward sex:

The church in the Middle Ages sentenced those who committed fornication to the same kind of punishments as those persons who were guilty of murder.

Holy men have often spread more than "The Word":

A Buddhist monk from Tibet introduced the artificial phallus to China. The monk appeared in the Imperial capital and presented Empress Wu Tse-tien's personal physician, Ming Ch'ung-yen, with a dildo. Wu Tse-tien (who ruled from A.D. 685–704), was extremely pleased to receive the dildo, which was made out of rubber and called "the live limb."

The church has often gone to great lengths to protect the sexual purity of its followers:

In the fourth century A.D., the Church did not even trust the dead to stay sexually honest. For this reason, the Second Council of Macon decreed that a female corpse had to be completely decomposed before a male could be buried beside her.

The work of the church in controlling the erotic desires of the "savage" has not been easy:

Catholic missionaries on the Marquesas Islands in the South Pacific had difficulty in keeping the sexes apart and uncoupled. One of the activities designed to occupy the Marquesas with thoughts other than sex was football, otherwise known as soccer. The missionaries thought that a good game of soccer would leave the natives too exhausted to indulge in sex. The Marquesas had a different point of view. They continually frustrated the supervising churchmen by making the game an opportunity to chase their desired partners well after the ball had gone to someone else. As a result, the game, stirring the blood of the natives, only encouraged them to pursue each other and frustrated the churchmen.

Missionaries on the Polynesian Islands often herded Polynesian boys into a large hut at night, so that the young men could not sneak out of their own huts in the middle of the night and have sex with the girls. Satisfied that they were preventing sin amongst the natives, the missionaries slept with a sense of satisfaction. However, they learned the next day that the boys, while not going out to meet the girls, had sex anyway. With each other.

Medical ignorance has at times caused humiliation for loyal church-fearing people:

In the 17th and 18th centuries in the United States, citizens were forbidden by the church to have sexual relations on Sundays. At the time, it was believed that babies were born on the same day of the week as they were created. For this reason, because couples were forbidden to have intercourse on Sunday, any child born on a Sunday was a product of sin and refused baptism.

The church has at times preached that love of a mate and love of God could not exist together:

During the Middle Ages, Malfre Ermengaud argued, "Satan, in order to make men suffer bitterly, makes them adore women; for instead of loving, as they should, the Creator, with fervent love, with all their heart, with all their mind and understanding, they sinfully love women, whom they make into deities. Know ye that whosoever adores them, doth most certainly adore Satan, and make a god of the most disloyal Devil, Belial."

Shame has been used to control the sexual impulses of the faithful:

Tertullian, the 3rd-century Christian Church father, said, "Do you realize, Eve, that...The curse God pronounced on your sex weighs still in the world. Guilty, you must bear its hardships. You are the Devil's gateway, you desecrated the fatal tree, you first betrayed the law of God, you softened up with your cajoling words the man against whom the Devil could not prevail by force. The image of God, Adam, you broke him as if he were a plaything. You deserved death, and it was the son of God who had to die!"

St. Bernard agreed with the use of shame to rule the flock: "Man is nothing else than a fetid sperm, a sack of dung, the food of worms. You have never seen a viler dung-hill."

There have been extreme restrictions on the appropriate time to have sex:

From the 7th to the 12th centuries, theologians determined to restrict the practice of sex severely.
   Tuesdays and Wednesdays, they suggested, were proper for lovemaking. Couples were to abstain on Thursdays, to observe the day that Christ was arrested. Friday sex was forbidden, because it was the day on which Christ died. Saturdays, chastity was required in honor of the

Virgin Mary. Sundays were disallowed for sex because that was the day of Christ's resurrection; Mondays, out of respect for the dead.

Very often, though, Tuesdays and Wednesdays were still restricted from sexual indulgence, if certain other occasions fell on those days. There was also a ban on intercourse during fasts and festivals, such as 40 days before Easter, Pentecost and Christmas, and various other occasions. This left the man and woman a handful of days in the whole year when it was acceptable to show sexual love.

The 7th-century abbot, Cummean Fota, wrote the penitential for couples of the time. Sexual abstinence was demanded of the couple for three different 40-day periods in the course of a year. Saturdays, Sundays, Wednesdays and Fridays were off limits as well. No sex was allowed during the woman's period. This left a total of about 81 days a year allowed for sexual conduct. Should the couple have had a child, this number was further reduced. They were not allowed to have sex for 33 days after the birth of a son or, interestingly, 66 days after the birth of a daughter. This could leave as few as 20 days per year for lovemaking.

☀

The church refused to recognize sex as an activity for pleasure and promoted it only as something for the purpose of creating children:

During the Middle Ages, sex, even within marriage, was considered by the church to be loathsome and sinful. Pleasure was not to be a part of sex; sex was only the undesirable means necessary to creating children. To discourage pleasure during the act, the church endorsed the use of the chemise cagoule.

The chemise cagoule allowed sex without encouraging passion or permitting too much titillation. The chemise cagoule was a long, thick, heavy woolen nightshirt worn by women, with a hole in the front to permit her partner penetration.

☀

Philo Judaeus (13 B.C.–A.D. 45) called those men who used contraceptives while having sex "effeminate" because they pursued "unnatural pleasure" and worked toward "the destruction and depopulation of the cities." The punishment for using contraceptives: "He should be killed without hesitation, and not be allowed to live a day, indeed not for an hour."

☀

Sex was painted in the ugliest of colors. The church encouraged guilt should anyone find sex pleasurable, even with the chemise cagoule. This "loathsome act" was the object of the pure person's disgust:

56

Oswald Cockayne wrote a scathing condemnation of sex in *Hali Maidenhead*, written in the Middle Ages. He not only disapproved of premarital sex, he found the married relation equally repulsive: "Into the filth of the flesh, into the manner of life of a beast, into thralldom of a man, and into the sorrows of the world...to cool thy lust with filth of thy body, to have delight of thy fleshly will from man's intercourse; before God, it is a nauseous thing to think thereon, and to speak thereof is yet more nauseous. Consider of what sort that thing itself, and that deed be done. All that foul delight is in filth ended, as thou turnest thy hand. But that loathesome beast remains and lasts on: and the disgust at long after."

Some representatives of the church were not satisfied with a limitation of times appropriate for sex, or the limit of physical contact:

Both Ambrose and Tertullian believed that if the only way to keep the human species alive was to have men and women endure the low and disgusting feelings and actions of intercourse, it would be better that the human race die out.

It was the Christian Church father St. Odon of Cluny who charmingly remarked, "We are born between shit and piss."

As severe as the church could be about the frequency or desirability of sex, it could show charity:

The cardinal Santa Lucia received and carried out the recommendation that he make sodomy legal for June, July and August of each year.

If the act itself could not be cast in an ugly light, the church encouraged its participants to be so:

Tertullian, third century A.D. ancient Roman church father, in the early days of the Christian Church, rejected all cosmetics and clothing which enhanced a woman's charms. He even suggested that the pure woman be careful to make herself ugly: "Even natural beauty ought to be obliterated by concealment and neglect, since it is dangerous to all who look upon it."

Religious art was not left untouched by the puritanism of the church:

In 1555, Michelangelo's frescoes on the ceiling of the Sistine Chapel were declared obscene. Pietro Aretino, a moralist of the time, brought pressure on Pope Paul IV to destroy the obscenities.

It was finally agreed that the nude figures in the religious fresco *The Last Judgment* would be covered with clothes. Daniele Volterra, a disciple of Michelangelo's, was commissioned to paint clothes onto the original characters. After doing so, his peers nicknamed Volterra Il Braghettone, or "The Breeches Maker."

Western religion has always believed that the physical was not compatible with the spiritual, even when it was successfully practiced:

The Picards of 16th-century France practiced "religious nudity," believing that the leader of their group had been sent as a "new Adam," and that as such, they should be "dressed" as Adam was. The Hussites did not agree with the Picards' philosophy, and for this, they slaughtered the Picards.

Europeans have often been horrified to discover what other religions considered holy:

New Mexican Navaho transvestites were highly regarded. These bardajes, called "nadle," were considered lucky, held in great esteem, and, as a result, were usually very wealthy.

At times the church encouraged the legal marriage of couples by declaring that they were, by intimate contact, already obligated to each other:

The archbishop Winchesley declared in 1308 that partners who fornicated three times instantly became legal man and wife as of their very first sexual contact.

The sexual organ played a religious role in attesting to the honor of men:

A member of Napoleon Bonaparte's army in Egypt in the 18th century noted the strange manner in which a man of the Mameluke tribe swore to his honor. In pleading innocence to being a spy, the Mameluke pledged his honor by solemn religious oath, while grasping his penis in hand.

Arabs swore on their genitals. Dervishes of the 19th-century Sudan asked that their organs fall off if they broke their solemn oath. Then they asked the persons to whom they pledged their honor to "take my seed into thy hand, that the vow be sealed forever."

Another oath was called the Oath of the Uncircumcised Penis. The men involved gave their word while holding each other's genitals.

The keepers of the faith frequently enjoyed privileges that they denied others:

The Catholic Church of the 1500s used castrated boys in their choirs. Women were not allowed to sing in churches, so Castrati, or Soprani, castrated boys, were used when high voices were needed. These desexed boys were chosen to be castrated at the age of six or seven. The church had always forbidden castration by all other people, under all other circumstances, but did not ban the use of Castrati in churches until Pope Leo XIII outlawed castration by the church in 1880.

In the early 17th century, these Soprani began to appear outside the church. This created a class of musical eunuchs called Evirati. These ex-choirboys became favorites of the stage and opera, and many of the desexed young men were the objects of female love. At least one, Tenducci, even married and lived happily with his wife.

Unfortunately, churchgoers sometimes found it necessary to protect themselves from the sin of adultery by endorsing it:

Concerned parishioners in medieval Switzerland and Spain sometimes ordered the local priest to take a mistress. This was, unfortunately, necessary to protect their own women from the clergyman's passions.

Germany's men of the cloth were no different:

The sexual behavior of the clergy in medieval Germany can be summed up in the word for "bastard." The word is *Praffenkind*, and it meant "parson's child."

Nor were Caribbean missionaries:

In 16th-century Bahai, the missionary priests were commonly addressed by their mistress's names.

In its history, the church has had to resort to very practical measures to restrain the sexual desires of monks and nuns:

In 1179 in Rome, a church council assembly, the Third Lateran Council, directed that a lamp burn in every convent dormitory at night.

As well, nuns were strictly forbidden to sleep together in the same bed. This was to curb the nuns' tendencies toward, as the council put it, "...incontinence which is against nature."

The monks and nuns ignored the warnings against homosexual activity. The Council of Paris in 1212 and the Council of Rouen (1214) had to repeat the prohibition and added more rules. Nuns could not be together in each other's rooms, and they had to leave their doors unlocked so that the abbess could check on them unannounced.

The holy man, while not allowing the sexual activities of his fellow man, found satisfaction where he could:

The medieval French Papal Legate had been faced with so many cases of priests involved in incest that priests were formally forbidden to live with relatives. This order was enforced and had to be repeated regularly, for more than 300 years.

In the 16th and 17th centuries, in Pescia, Italy, the Franciscan monks socialized regularly with the nuns. The nuns of Santa Chiara enjoyed their company so much that in 1610 the Provost of Santa Chiara confronted the fornicating friars. The nuns were so angered by the possibility of losing their lovers that they pelted the Provost's men with bricks and stones, chasing them off.

The Incas had a stable of young religious girls, called the Virgins of the Sun. These young women, nuns of a sort, swore themselves to chastity at risk of death. The only acceptable explanation for an unexpected pregnancy was to claim the father of the child to be the sun, in which case she was spared the penalty of being burned alive.

Normally, deviant sexual behavior, even necrophilia, has sometimes been required of a holy man in fulfilling his duties:

In ancient Egypt, no female was allowed to be buried as a virgin. In the case of the death of a girl premature to losing her virginity, the dead girl was sexually embraced by the embalmer or the priest.

In the service of preaching to their followers, holy men have used unorthodox methods of getting their point across:

The people of Syracuse, in ancient Greece, often made an offering to the gods consisting of little cakes shaped to resemble the women's vulva. A priest, practicing ventriloquism, persuaded the crowd that the vulva cakes were speaking, making holy pronouncements.

It has not been uncommon for the religious institution to put financial interest ahead of concern for sexual morality:

In London in February of 1790, a woman in Swadlincote was abandoned by her husband. In financial distress, she had to rely on the charity of the parish. The head of the parish, to relieve the financial obligation, sold the woman at Burton Market to a man. The parish received one florin from her new master.

The prohibition against women socially associating with others while they had their period has been a feature of tribal peoples. The Christian Church agreed with the aboriginal philosophy in the not-so-distant past:

The medieval church considered it a sin if a woman went to church while she had her period.

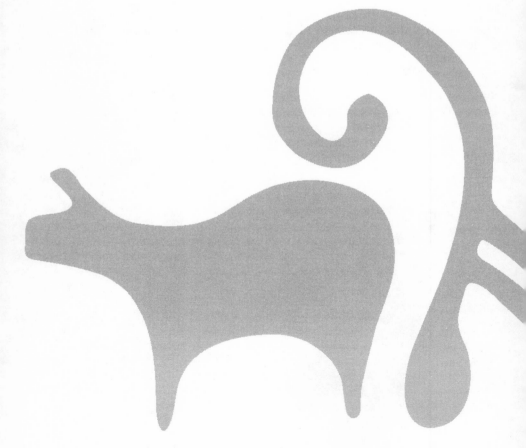

SEX EDUCATION—
ROOTS

Some of the origins of words shed a very different light on the nature of the word:

The Greek word for a sexual romp, *orgy*, was originally a word that referred to religious ceremonies.

The word *whore* has ancient beginnings. The Celts called their sexual businesswomen Cara, the ancient Norse Hora. The Anglo-Saxon word was *Hore-cwen.*

These words were probably derived from the Indo-European *car.* Later on amongst the Anglo Saxons, *Hore-cwen* was the source of the word *cwen*, or "queen."

Phallus is a Greek word derived from the Latin *fascinium*, which meant "magical spirit." The word *fascinate* is related to both *phallus* and *fascinium*, but a preoccupation with the male organ, or its mesmerizing power, is now rarely associated with the common use of the word *fascinate.*

The ancient Greeks coined the term *virgo*, which is the modern-day "virgin." However, this term had originally applied only to women, because the meaning of *virgo* is "a girl or woman not known by a man."

During the reign of Charles I of England, an unmarried English actress was usually addressed as "Mistress" (no doubt because so many of them entertained married lovers). Later it was shortened, and the title changed in meaning. The unmarried girl was called "Miss," and its new meaning was commonly understood as "concubine."

The word *testicle* comes from the Latin words *testiculi* and *testes*, meaning "witnesses." They were considered the witnesses to the procreative act.

The Arab word *harem* or *harim* does not take the meaning which other cultures may attach to it. It was not considered a "prison" or anything of the kind. The meaning of *harem* is "(woman's) sanctuary."

The application of certain words has changed since their introduction. For instance, a glamorous girl in the 16th and 17th centuries was burned at the stake. The word *glamor* comes from the time of the Spanish Inquisition. A woman who was thought to be a witch cast a bewitching look, or "glamor."

Other word origins:

The English name for the fifth day of the week, Friday, is a descendant of the Anglo-Saxon *Frige-daeg*, which descended from the ancient *Friga*. Friga was the goddess of love and sex.

The Gnostics and Manicheans were harassed by and persecuted as heretics by the Catholic Church. Many of these people took refuge in Bulgara. These religious outlaws (as was the custom of the propagandists of the church) were accused of sodomy. The French called these people Bolgres, or Bogres. The name stuck and took on the meaning of "sodomite." The term *bugger* is still used to mean "a sodomite" or "sodomy," all these centuries later.

The ancient Greek word *hexis* may be the origin of the word *sex*. The Greeks called man's moral and physical state hexis.

The word *sex* may owe its existence to the Roman *secare*, "to cut or sever," or *sexus*, "the difference between men and women."

The word *bordello* (whorehouse), originated in medieval France. The French whorehouse was considered a small house of boards, or bordel. It was inhabited by a whore, or brothel, from whence came the other term for whorehouse, *brother*.

The ancient Romans are responsible for the word *masturbate*. Their term for the act was *manusturbo*, "to defile with the hands."

The ancient Romans equated the left hand with crudeness and impropriety. The latin word for left meant "sinister," and there was an aversion to the left hand. It was in this way that the left hand was associated with the practice of masturbation.

The word *taboo*, which frequently takes on a sexual meaning, originated with the Polynesians. When a woman was menstruating, she was considered tapu, or "off limits."

Ancient Greece is the first known source of a word to designate a homosexual person. These people, males, were known as *paiderastes*, or "boy-lovers." The word later was transformed as "pederast," and for a very long time after this practice in ancient Greece, although these homosexuals were not necessarily involved with boys, the term *pederast* was the only term used to describe homosexuals.

The term *gonorrhea* was coined in ancient Rome by a Greek physician. Its meaning gives a very vivid image of the consequences of the illness. *Gonorrhea*, means, very literally, "the flow of seed."

The courtesan was a highly paid Italian whore who was kept by a select number of very generous clients: usually well moneyed and well titled. The term *courtesan* is believed to have come from *cortesia*, or "courtesy." Thus, her business was more refined than that of the common prostitute: She merely received the "courtesies" of her select "friends."

The Greek word *syphilis* means "swine" and "love"; a very obvious reference to the belief of the source from which this disease came.

Later, in 1530, the Italian Girolamo Fracastoro wrote a poem about the origin of syphilis. Syphilis was a Greek shepherd who had been punished by Apollo with the disease because he practiced unnatural intercourse.

The concept of chastity is truly a religious one. The Greeks called the "chaste," or sexually unspoiled, Castus. Loosely translated, this means "adhering to the religious way."

Eunuchs were employed as domestic help in the Far East. Eunuchs were the only male servants trusted to wait on their master's wives, since they were castrated. *Eunuch*, the term used to describe the castrated manservant, meant "chamberlain," or, more clearly, "belonging to the bedchamber."

In the Middle and Far East, the word *tent* was used as the synonym for a woman.

The name for woman in Arabic was *orett*. It also meant "nakedness" and "shame."

The Tahitian word for menstrual blood was *vari*—which also meant "mud."

Arabs called lesbians who had overdeveloped clitorises (capable of visible erection) Bazar. This word also translates as "slut," or "wench."

A common term for venereal disease, coined in England, was *the clap*. This was an abbreviated form of "the disease I picked up while I was clapped together with someone."

The word *aphrodisiac* is derived from the ancient Roman festival of Aphrodisia, Goddess of Love. It was here that some of the earliest aphrodisiacs—both potions and love charms—were sold and used.

It was St. Augustine who termed the genitals *pudenda*, or "shameful parts." He labeled them so because mankind was ashamed that these parts were the only ones he had no control over. Interestingly enough, it is common that *pudenda* is usually used only in reference to women's genitals.

Prostitute is derived from the Latin word *putaeus*, the Latin connotation of the word being "tank," or "spring." Thus, a prostitute was a spring from which all men could drink.

Obscenities have very old beginnings:

The Latin *fornication* was changed to *Vokken* in low German. About 1735, *Fokken*—"to breed"—made its appearance in language. The word underwent another change, to *Ficken*, before making its way into the English language as *Fuck*.

The crude term *cunt* has undergone many transformations. In Old English it was *Queynt*: previously it was *Cunnus*, from the ancient Greeks. But its very root is much older than that. The granddaddy of the English language, Sanskrit, named the female part *Cushi*, or "waterditch."

The term *fetish* is derived from the Greek word *facere*, or "to fascinate."

The meaning of the word *castrate* is found in the 15th-century work *Hortus Sanitatis*. In it, the behavior of the beaver (Latin: *castor*) was described. If vigorously pursued, it claimed, the beaver, or castor, bit off his reproductive organs and left them for the pursuer. If further followed, the castor stood up on his hind legs and showed the persistent follower his lack of genitals.

The early Anglo-Saxons were responsible for the word *wed*. A wed was a dowry that the groom gave to the bride's father. Often, the wed was given by the groom's father as proof of his ability to support the couple.

The word *honeymoon* comes from a custom originating in northern Europe. For a full month—or moon—after the wedding, the couple drank mead. Mead was a wine made of honey—thus, "honeymoon."

The custom of having a "best man" at a wedding is very old, though the birthdate of the custom is unknown. It is thought that originally the best man was the friend most fit to help the groom capture the bride, at a time when marriage by abduction or pretended abduction was the custom.

The best man was usually called on to hold off, either in real style or mock fighting fashion, the family members who came to the bride's rescue. The aspect of capturing the bride has, for the most part, disappeared, but the tradition continues.

SEX EDUCATION—
RECIPES

In ancient cultures, menstrual blood was thought to be a potent substance:

In ancient Egypt, menstruation and menstrual blood were regarded with repulsion. It was believed that when mixed with other substances, with the moon in the proper place, mentrual blood became the active ingredient in poison. This poison supposedly slowly killed its victim, and there was no antidote.

In some places, it was believed that food had the power to influence desires:

A very old love potion prevailed among peasants in the area of what is now Czechoslovakia. A lovesick person made the object of their desire fall in love with them by presenting them with a little cake. One of the ingredients of this cake was hair from the giver's armpit.

The Lepch people were convinced that eating uncastrated pigs would turn them into homosexuals. They believed that if a man happened to eat the flesh of an uncastrated pig, he would afterward desire to commit sodomy. To commit sodomy, or Nam-toak, also resulted in the offender suffering a year of misfortune.

To curb the sexual appetite, the ancient Greeks used several medicines:

The Greek scholar and historian Pliny the Elder (A.D. 23–79) had several recipes for curbing the sexual inclination. One of these was the application of a liniment made of mouse dung.

A cure for the desire for sex, one that was taken orally by the Greeks, consisted of oil, wine and snail or pigeon droppings.

Another solution to amativeness was to conceal the blood and testicles of a dunghill cock under the marriage bed.

A fourth method of cooling the passions, on the part of the woman, was the rubbing of her loins with the blood of ticks taken off the back of a black bull.

Restoring the sexual vigor has been the concern of many worried couples. Many have fallen prey to dubiously "scientific" doctors with "surefire" cures:

A medical charlatan, the Scot Dr. James Graham, had a very fashionable spa in the 1780s. He was famous for his elixirs and exercises that supposedly cured sexual ills. These were to be found in his "Temple of Health." He invented the graham cracker as a biscuit that would satisfy the hunger without inflaming the passions.

A bedchamber called the Oriental Celestial Bed was rented out to troubled couples who were in search of sexual vigor. For 50 English pounds per night, the couple occupied the bed, which was supported by 28 glass pillars and was canopied.

The more civilized of cultures have often followed the example of their more primitive brothers in believing in the medicinal value of human by-products:

In ancient Greece and also in Rome, a man suffering from impotence was prescribed a tonic of animal semen.

In many parts of Australia, the aborigines gave their very sick or dying medicine in the form of semen.

As recently as the 17th century in England, urine was frequently used as a medicine.

Recipes for the enlargement of the male member:

Advice from an ancient Arab text: To increase the size of the male sexual parts, a man was to boil the penis of an ass, along with corn and onions. One fed this preparation to the chickens, and then fed on the chickens himself.

To enlarge the male organ, the Japanese man went to the baths. There he could obtain a hot brick with a hole in it. To increase the circumference of his organ, he was instructed to put his penis through this hole.

In some parts of the world, and at various times in history, small breasts have been popularly attractive:

The recipe for the reduction of breasts, or their curtailment, from *Bastiment des Receptes:* Mince the heart, liver, lungs and spleen of a rabbit. Mix in the same amount of honey. Apply it to the breasts and chest area. When dry, apply another coating.

The Chinese believed that by binding the feet of their women, the female's thighs and vaginas were rendered more suitable and pleasing for intercourse, and in fact, the women who had their feet bound were found to have more fully developed parts than their neighbors, the Tartar women.

Sometimes very simple procedures could yield great results:

In England in the 19th century, it was believed that women who had the nipples of their breasts pierced had fuller, rounder bosoms than others.

The Arab man valued his potency and was willing to accept help in this area:

A two-part cure for sterility: On a piece of linen, place the marrow from a camel's hump. Rub the linen cloth over the genitals consistently. At the same time, fast for seven days, drinking only the juice of the "Jackal's Grapes," mixed with vinegar. And, of course, the man should give his lover all his attention.

To prolong the sex drive, we need look no further than the ancient Middle East, which produced several cookbooks of love:

The recipe for sexual strength, according to the author of *The Perfumed Garden,* written in the 14th century: "The fruit of the mastic tree is mashed and oil and honey are added. The liquid product is then consumed as soon as one rises in the morning."

Sexual vigor for males and females could be attained by rubbing the genitals with the fluid from the liver of a jackal.

To prolong their potence, keeping the sexual life active, men rubbed their penises with ass's milk.

The ancient Hebrew woman accused of adultery was put to a test. Her husband escorted her to the temple with a small quantity of barley meal. The priest brought her a jug of water. She took the barley meal into her hands and said "Yahweh." She drank the water and ate some dust. If her stomach did not swell up, she was pronounced innocent; if it swelled, she was considered guilty of adultery.

Hottentot women, on seeing the rain fall, took off all their clothes and ran into the rain, because they believed that the rain would make them, like the ground, fertile.

Women of the northern Gold Coast, to increase their fertility, engaged in sex with animals.

For some men and women, precautions were taken when they were born to assure their sexual charms:

In 17th-century England it was a common practice for the midwives to take special care in cutting the umbilical cord. In the case of boys, the cord was cut as long as possible, to enhance his penis length. The "navel-cord" of female babies was cut as short as possible to enhance the narrowness of their vaginas.

Providing for the health of an infant could be an enjoyable responsibility:

The eastern Bolivian Sironos practiced frequent intercourse once a woman was pregnant. The additional installments of semen, they believed, made the baby grow larger and larger.

Among many cultures, sexual intercourse was considered healthy. Others have preached the ill effects of not indulging:

At the time of the Gunabibi festival, all Murngin men and women were obligated to practice free love with the rest of their tribe. It was believed that unrestrained intercourse at this time purified the body, and to abstain would make a man or woman ill.

Among many of the old cultures, cleanliness of the sexual organs was carefully observed:

The ancient Egyptians practiced a unique form of hygiene. The Berin

Papyrus suggested regular fumigation of the anus and vagina. A liquid mixture was poured over hot coals while the man or woman squatted, catching the steaming fumes in the anus or vagina.

Women were advised to fumigate their vaginas in this manner to keep the womb from "wandering." It was thought that through regular airing of the vagina, the womb would return to its "natural place." The woman stood over hot coals, legs spread, while an ibis made of wax was placed on the hot coals at her feet.

Cures could involve the sacrifice of another person for the sake of a more "valuable" person:

The official physician to the rich and famous of Europe in the Middle Ages, including Cesare Borgia and Pope Alexander VI, was Bishop Tornella. During the great European syphilis epidemic of 1495–1503, Tornella's treatment for syphilis was to have a person of "low condition" suck the pus out of the patient's most severe syphilitic sore. This was usually on the genitals. The poor underling was considered disposable, and after his role in removing the pus of the sore was done, he was soon forgotten.

After some time, it appeared that the treatment wasn't working. Tornella's next procedure was more elaborate. He cut open the belly of a mule, taking care to make sure it stayed alive. He then lowered the patient into the still warm, live mule's belly.

One of the first institutions to treat venereal diseases was located in England. In 13th-century London, Lock Hospital made a specialty of treating the venereally afflicted. The treatments: washing with roses and herbs boiled in vinegar, running, jumping, inhaling pepper, and in the case of women, tickling the vagina with a feather.

While venereal disease has long been a problem, in some instances it was believed to be a solution:

In medieval England, during the time of the Plague, or Black Death, it was believed that the only way to prevent getting the Plague was to have venereal disease. Doctors thought that anyone with syphilis or gonorrhea was immune to the Black Death.

Fertility has always been a primary sexual concern:

Women of the Adaman Islands ensured fertility by making a stew of frogs.

The folk custom of Estonian brides who were seeking to bear children was to eat a meal of goat testicles.

Every year in January, Indian women of the tribes of Coimbatore, Kara-madai and Jungingatta committed themselves to having sex with a certain number of men, all strangers, at a fertility festival. In this way they were made more fertile.

In Kurdistan, among the Dusiks, certain fertility was ensured shortly after marriage to one lucky bride. At the yearly festival, the most recent bride was rendered fertile by the holy man of the temple. All people gathered, then the resident holy man proclaimed, "I am the Great Bull!" The most recently married girl stepped forward and proclaimed, "I am the Young Cow!" After this proclamation, they had intercourse, which was followed by intercourse among the other members of the temple.

The irresistible cravings of pregnant women have been termed *pica*. This condition has been cured by the woman indulging herself in her cravings. This craving can and has gone to extremes. In one account from 1725, a woman from Italy ate several pounds of sand and topped it off with a glass of her own urine.

The Riffian boys of northwest coastal Africa developed their sexual powers and strengthened their penises by having sex with female asses.

SEX EDUCATION—
THEORIES AND PHILOSOPHIES

Sexual scientists have spent a lifetime studying sex and culture. There have been some curious theories put forth by often poorly qualified sexologists:

Sir Richard Burton, traveler of Africa and the Middle East for 30 years, believed that geography determined sexual appetite. He observed that men were more passionate in countries with colder climates than females were. Women were supposedly more sexually ardent than men in "warm, damp countries lying close to mountains."

The symbolism of the vagina as devouring the penis is present in most societies, to a greater or lesser degree:

The Cayapan Indians of southern Ecuador referred to sexual intercourse as "the vagina eating the penis." These men considered this very literally, and for this reason had a great fear of intercourse.

Some sexual scientists believed that the seasons determined the frequency of intercourse desired:

Pythagoras, 6th-century B.C. Greek philosopher and mathematician, believed that there were seasons favorable for intercourse. He taught his students that indulging in sex in the winter was healthful. In the spring and fall, it was not harmful but was to be avoided whenever possible. Summer, he claimed, was not the season for the reproductive act, and summertime sex should be abstained from.

There have been other strange medical theories put forth:

The ancient Greeks and Romans believed that all of a woman's health problems could be cured by treating her genitals, as her reproductive organs were the source of all her suffering.

It only made sense, then, that a girl should be married by puberty, so that by "using" her organs of reproduction, these diseases would be stopped.

One of the most common of these was hysteria. A woman's womb was believed to wander through the body. Hysteria would result if the womb could not make its way back to the vagina. The cure for hysteria, then, was to lure the womb back to the vagina. This was done by inserting sweet-smelling substances into an hysterical girl's vagina. The womb, attracted by the sweet smell, made its way "home."

The Roman physician Galen believed that once the blood had circulated throughout the male's body, it turned white and ended its journey in the testicles, as sperm.

In 1666 a German doctor, Sigmund Elsholz, suggested that marriages could be made happier if spouses of different temperaments exchanged blood. He believed that by a "hot-blooded" husband giving some of his blood to his "cold-blooded" wife (or vice versa), and receiving some of hers in return, their tempers would even out each other.

The ancient Greek Eustathius reported that Amazons were in the habit of taking their war prisoners and breaking their limbs. This was not to prevent the captives from escaping. Rather, the Amazons thought it beneficial for their population to have prisoners have intercourse with their women, and also believed that for the male sexual limb to be vigorous, it was best that other limbs did not sap its strength.

The Murngin people, in celebrating the Gunabibi festival, exchanged partners freely and frequently. However, after each encounter with a strange woman, the man "protected" himself from sickness. This was done by "baptizing" the lover. The woman's husband smeared some of his sweat over his wife's lover's arms and legs.

In Europe in the Middle Ages, it was suggested that moderate sexual contact with young boys was good for a man's health.

Moslems made it taboo to have intercourse during a woman's period. The belief was that sex during her period would cause leprosy.

The natives of the Marquesas Islands believed that men could "cure" an unusually long menstrual period by having sex with the woman.

The East African Bantu man of the Akambas could have sexual intercourse at any time he desired, with one exception: He was always obligated to have sex with his wife on the first day of her period. The

Akamba believed that the most fertile time for intercourse was the first day of a woman's period, and thus, it was the man's duty to perform.

An East African Nandi man bitten by a snake cured the effects of the poison by speeding up the circulation of his blood. The remedy for snake bites, then, was sex.

In the early 19th century in England, females suffering from chlorosis (also called "green sickness"), in an effort to cure the illness, were advised by doctors to masturbate with turkey necks.

The Aborigines of Australia removed the clitoris from every female of the tribe. This was done because it was believed that left to itself, it would sprout "shoots" and continue to grow in every direction.

Old Arab medical books considered the taking of a girl's virginity a cure for many ills. It was considered a sure cure for any male suffering from depression, melancholy and impotence, among other things.

The use of medical misinformation to justify morals or sexual tastes has been widespread:

Ainu women were taught to lay absolutely still during intercourse; otherwise, their husbands would suffer misfortune and die very poor.

The sexually uninhibited Mohaves of New Mexico had one sexual practice that was not indulged in. Mohave men disliked the way their women smelled—particularly their genitals. They refused to practice cunnilingus, as they believed that if the man's face came too close to the vagina, he would go blind.

Superstition has played a very large part in sex—the sexual act being very mysterious in many cultures:

Among the East African Waccamba and Wacicuga tribes, intercourse was forbidden while the cows were in the pastures.

Witches and sorcerers were, in the 16th century, blamed for many sexual ills. Women who could not conceive blamed the spell-casters. Men who could not gain erection looked about them for the witch who had cursed them in this way.

In France, the lovesick man, in an effort to win a girl's heart, wore a swallow's heart tied to his penis.

While the male sexual organ has nearly always been considered lucky, the opposite is generally true of the female genitals:

In ancient Rome, the phallic image could be seen everywhere. It dominated styles of jewelry, and it was seen on chariots and on soldier's armor. Bakers, advertising their fertility value, baked phallic-shaped breads, cookies and cakes. The phallic symbol was placed above doorways of shops and homes, and in gardens to help the flowers, bushes and trees grow. There was no place in which the phallus was not used to bring fertility and thus good fortune.

In ancient Greece, a gold or coral sculpture of a penis was worn by people as a good-luck charm. It protected against witchcraft and especially against the Evil Eye.

In ancient Greece and into the Middle Ages in Europe, curious objects were sold on festive occasions. At the Italian festivals of the Holy Cosismus and Damianus, peddlers sold wax phalluses.

In parts of China, it was considered bad fortune for the male to see the female's genitals—particularly first thing in the morning.

There have been exceptions to this rule, however:

Neapolitan Italians used to protect themselves against the Jettatori, or spell-casters, with the Sign of the Fig. This was made by pushing the thumb through the space between the index finger and the middle finger. This symbolized the female sexual parts and prevented a spell from being effective against the person who made the sign.

The Kamba of the African coast hunted sea lions. It was believed that the hunter would be dragged into the ocean on the next hunt if he did not have sex with the sea cow he killed.

In Germany, a woman desiring a certain man prepared a "love potion" by going to bed with an apple or biscuit in her vagina. The next day she presented it to the man of her choice, and once eaten, he fell in love with her.

It is an ageless belief that a well-endowed male is a good provider and fighter:

The Roman general Heliogabalus believed that men with large noses also had large penises and were thus considered superior fighters. The 18th-century sexologist Nicolas Venette says that Heliogabalus chose "Big nosed Soldiers, that he might be able to undertake great Expeditions with small Numbers, and oppose his Enemy with greater vigour."

However, Venette voiced an objection to this preference: "At the same time he did not take notice, that well hung Men are the greatest Blockheads, and the most stupid of Mankind."

There has been much variance, between cultures and across time, in the beliefs of the sexual nature of women. There have been as many sources claiming women to be naturally frigid as there were experts claiming them to be of hot temper:

Venette believed women to be of passionate temper and were the worse off for it: "They are much more amorous than Men; and as Sparrows do not live long, because they are too hot, and too susceptible of love, so Women last less time; because they have a devouring heat that consumes them by degrees."

The ancient Chinese were convinced of the ability of women to pass the gift of fertility from themselves to men:

The Taoist Chinese cure for impotence was to have the affected man touch his tongue and lips to the vulva of a very passionate girl. He then performed cunnilingus upon her until she reached orgasm. It was vital that the impotent man swallow all her orgasmic secretions.

The amorous nature has been attributed to some unlikely sources:

The Roman physician Oribasius believed that chickpeas, vaccet onions, broad beans, pine kernels, octopus and flax seeds made men more amorous because they were foods that produced flatulence. Oribasius believed that these "gassy" foods were ideal because they made the sperm "froth."

That the sexual urge is strong is very evident in the fact that many cultures view the erotic impulse as out of one's control:

The Cayapans of Ecuador did not consider sexual relations a matter of choice. Their explanation for the procreative urge was that "when the penis wants to bother a woman, it erects itself."

The punishment for supposedly improper behavior could be very harsh:

When missionaries followed the Conquistadors into Mexico to convert the Mexicans, they were horrified at the sexual practices of the natives. Because they practiced homosexuality, bestiality, masturbation and sexual positions not approved of by the church, missionaries had a huge "re-educating" job before them.

Thus, they told the Mexicans that because they practiced homosexuality, bestiality and masturbation, God had sent the Conquistadors (who had done an efficient job of slaughtering these people) to punish them.

Among many peoples, reproduction was less than clearly understood:

The ancient Greek doctors believed that the nose and lungs of a woman were an important part of her reproductive system. They believed that a woman's breathing and her breeding parts worked closely together in creating a child. Often, a woman was tested for fertility by placing substances, such as garlic, in her vagina. If after 12 hours the woman could "breathe" this substance out of her mouth, it was thought that she would be good at reproducing.

The Trobriand Island people believed that man had no role in reproduction. The creation of the child was believed to be accomplished by the woman and the spirit. For this reason, males had no claims over their wives or children.

Women and girls of lower Brittany were told not to look at the moon while urinating. The belief was that if they did so, they would become "moonstruck"—pregnant from the motion of the moon. This would cause them to give birth to a moon-child, or "lunatic."

Among the Tully River tribe (Queensland, Australia), men and women believed that a man impregnated a woman when he passed a roasted fish over the fire to the woman.

Some tribes of Polynesia believed that a girl would not become pregnant as long as she often changed sexual partners.

In an effort at sexual variance, theory has often seemed to eclipse the practical side of the sexual possibility:

The Kamasutra, the ancient Indian love manual, describes many variations of sexual position. A great number of these, however, are possible only for the extremely limber, or for contortionists. Such a position was called "Fixing of a Nail." The woman, while standing on one leg, received the man, while the foot of her other leg was on her head.

It appears that there was little that escaped the thoughtful minds of eroticists:

The East Indian erotic manual, *The Perfumed Garden*, was written by Shaykh Nefzawi in the 16th century. In it, many aspects of sex were discussed, including sex for hunchbacked individuals. In it he discussed sex between the hunched male and the normal female, the crooked female and healthy man, and intercourse between two hunchbacked partners. Included were six comfortable positions.

One of the greatest curiosities mankind has is for the sexual differences between peoples:

In ancient China, it was believed that women of different regions had differently shaped vaginas. The women most talked about were those of the Shansi Province, in Tantung county. These women were widely rumored to have had "double door" vaginas.

Sex has not been so complicated for others. In some cases, the how and the why were made very simple:

The Mohammedan philosophy of sex was that of the male master and the female servant. Passion and impulse ruled the relation of a man to his wife: "Your wives are your tillage; go therefore into your tillage in what manner soever you will."

A society's attitude toward sex is indicated by its language and reveals the values and morals of that society by its words:

In the 16th century, the French used more than 300 different words to refer to intercourse. They also used over 400 different words to refer to the male and female sexual organs.

In other places, the sexual act was expressed in the simplest and most common terms:

The Sumerians, who lived around 4000 B.C., described sex as "putting the hot fish in her navel."

Sexologists from all ages believed that there were tests to find out the sexual status of women. Distinguishing the virgin from the experienced girl was done in many ways:

Scotus determined virgins by studying their noses. In feeling the tips of their noses, he claimed that girls who had a division in the cartilage of their noses were virgins. Experienced women, however, had no cleave on the tips of their noses.

Musitano of Naples had a related theory: "Take a thread folded double, encircle the neck, mark the point which indicates the measure, and make a knot. After this, open out the second loop of thread so as to make one circle: if the head does not pass through, a woman is a virgin."

The feet were used by a certain Dr. Chavernac to identify virgins. They, he claimed, had feet that pointed straight forward. A nonvirgin, however, had feet that were definitely and permanently spread, pointing outward.

Further, he claimed he could tell if the woman had a left-handed or right-handed lover. If left-handed, the woman's left foot would be turned out farther than her right foot. However, because a right-handed man would tend to lay on the woman's right, her right foot would be turned out moreso than her left.

The Greek philosopher Virgil (70–19 B.C.), in Book Four of *Georgics*, had a method for determining virgins from nonvirgins. Bees, according to Virgil, would not attack a virgin, but would quite willingly attack an experienced woman. This was, he reasoned, because bees did not reproduce through sex, so naturally would have a horror of the being who showed signs of having had sex.

A doctor named Forestier believed that inhaling the smell of the patience plant (European Dock), when thrown on hot coals, could determine virginity. Upon smelling the plant on the hot coals, a virgin would supposedly urinate immediately and involuntarily.

William of Saliceto, a physician of the 13th century, theorized:

"A virgin urinates with a more subtle hiss than a nonvirgin; it takes her longer to finish than it does a small boy."

A woman's sexual capacity could be determined by her physical appearance:

The ancient Romans desired a very certain kind of woman. She had to be strong but not masculine. A woman had to look very feminine without being weak. A woman who blushed easily or whose face colored easily in anger was unsuitable; these women were of such hot constitution and desire that the male's semen would be "cooked."

Erotic objects date from the time of the caveman. Certain areas of the world have yielded ancient sexual objects. These artifacts were either fertility charms or erotic art:

The earliest recognizable erotic objects in existence were found in

France, the Ukraine and Siberia. These are small, chiseled-rock figures of Venus—the feminine ideal of the time. They are rock carvings of very fat women with large breasts and accentuated vulvae. These erotic figures have been dated as being more than 20,000 years old.

Sexual literature has been in existence since the time of the first attempts at keeping records:

Around 1300 B.C. the ancient Egyptians produced a work called the *Papyrus of Turin*. In it are diagrams and caricatures of men and women engaging in sex. There are 14 positions illustrated in this ancient erotic manual.

The art of erotic instruction has made lavish use of nature and language to explain the function:

Ars Amatoria, an ancient Chinese book of love, listed some very exotic positions for intercourse: Close Union, Firm Attachment, Exposed Gills, the Unicorn's Horn, Winding Dragon Position, Mandarin Ducks, Bamboos by the Altar, Cleaving Cicada, Phoenix Sporting in the Cinnabar Cleft, Gamboling Wild Horses, Hovering Butterflies.

The romance of erotic instruction was a feature of ancient Chinese sexual life:

Master Tung-hsuan, the author of *Ars Amatoria*, described one method of lovemaking: "The Jade Stalk should hover lightly around the entrance of the Cinnabar Gate while its owner kisses the woman lovingly or allows his eyes to linger over her body or look down upon her Golden Cleft. He should stroke her stomach and breasts and Jewel Entrance.

"As her desire increases, he should begin to move his Positive Peak more decisively, back and forward, bringing it now into direct contact with the Golden Cleft and Jade Veins, playing from side to side of the Examination Hall, and finally bringing it to rest at one side of the Jewel Entrance. Then when the Cinnabar Cleft is in flood, it is time for the Vigorous Peak to thrust forward."

In some cultures, sex did not have its own designation, but was more of a concept:

The Mangaian tribesmen of the Polynesian Islands had no specific term for the act of sex to orgasm; instead, it was called "the achievement of perfection."

In the ancient Middle East and India, the male genitals were carefully designated according to appearance and performance. *The Perfumed Garden* listed every kind of male organ a woman might encounter:

Sundry Names Given to the Sexual Parts of Man:

El air (The smith's bellows)
El hamma (The pigeon)
El teunnana (The tinkler)
El heurmak (The indomitable)
El ahil (The liberator)
El zeub (The verge)
El harmache (The exciter)
El naasse (The sleeper)
El zoddame (The crowbar)
El khiate (The turnabout)
Mochefi el reli (The extinguisher of passion)
El khorrate (The turnabout)
El deukkak (The striker)
El aouame (The swimmer)
El dekhal (The housebreaker)
El aaouar (The one-eyed)
El fortass (The bald one)
Abou aine (He with one eye)
El atsar (The stumbler)
El dommar (The odd-headed)
Abou rokba (The one with a neck)
Abou guetaia (The hairy one)
El besiss (The impudent)
El mostahi (The shamefaced)
El bekkai (The weeper)
El hezzaz (The rummager)
El lezzaz (The unionist)
Abou laaba (The expectorant)
El fattache (The searcher)
El hakkak (The rubber)
El mourekhi (The flabby one)
El motela (The ransacker)
El mokcheuf (The discoverer)

Other cultures were less particular concerning the manly organ:

Ancient Persians distinguished the manly endowment by one of two words. A man was either a *Zukkur* (carrot) or a *Keer* (worm).

Medieval Arabs believed women to be as sexually interested as men, if not moreso. An old Arab saying, concerning the sexual desires of women, went like this: "The Moslem woman prefers an additional inch of penis to anything this world or the next might offer."

The Perfumed Garden gave equal space to women and their particular kinds of sexual parts:

Sundry Names Given to the Sexual Organs of Women:

El feurdj (The slit)
El keuss (The vulva)
El relmoune (The voluptuous)
El ass (The primitive)
El zerzour (The starling)
El cheukk (The chink)
Abou tertour (The crested one)
Abou khochime (The snubnose)
El gueunfond (The hedgehog)
El sakouti (The silent one)
El deukkak (The crusher)
El tseguil (The importunate)
El taleb (The yearning one)
El hacene (The beautiful)
El neuffakh (The swelling one)
Abou djbaha (One with a projection)
El ouasa (The vast one)
El aride (The large one)
Abou belaoum (The glutton)
El mokaour (The bottomless)
Abou cheufrine (The two-lipped)
Abou aungra (The humpbacked)
El rorbal (The seive)
El lezzaz (The unionist)
El moudd (The accommodating)
El mouaine (The assistant)
El meusbou (The long one)
El molki (The duellist)
El harrab (The fugitive)
El sabeur (The resigned)
El mouseuffah (The barred one)
El merour (The deep one)
El addad (The biter)
El meusass (The sucker)
El zeunbour (The wasp)

El harr (The hot one)
El ladid (The delicious)

Designating the different natures of womens' sexual parts may have been useful, but her nature was universal:

Medieval Arab men considered women sexually insatiable:

"Who can stem a furious stream and a frantic woman? When in her recurrent frenzy of heat, man cannot appease her. It is like trying to stuff a bladder, with the essence oozing out the other end."

That women were slaves of their sexual capacity was "proved" medically:

The most commonly recognized female disease through the ages was hysteria. The disease was supposedly caused by a woman's physical need to reproduce. If this need was not satisfied, her body revolted. The ancient Greeks and Romans believed that a girl unmarried at the time of puberty had a womb that was not "open" because of lack of intercourse. The womb, then, would not allow blood to flow into it. This blood, flowing more fiercely now because it had not been allowed to go the proper route, rushed back to the girl's heart and diaphragm. Congestion and inflammation set in; delirium, fever, then lascivious desires appeared. The woman was overcome by her body's frustrated desire for sexual intercourse.

While women of the East were assumed to be more than willing participants in sex, in Europe women were thought to be less sexually inclined. Lovemaking technique reflected this belief:

In *De Regimine Sanitatis* (circa 1300), Arnoldus de Villanova described successful lovemaking of the time: First, the man started by caressing the woman's breasts. This, he warned, was to be attempted only when the woman was in the first stages of falling asleep. In this way, her natural shyness was overcome by tiredness.

Next, he suggested, the male waited until her "natural heat level" was "raised to a fever pitch." Then she was ready to be entered. The man would know when she was ready to be taken, said Arnoldus, when she started to "babble."

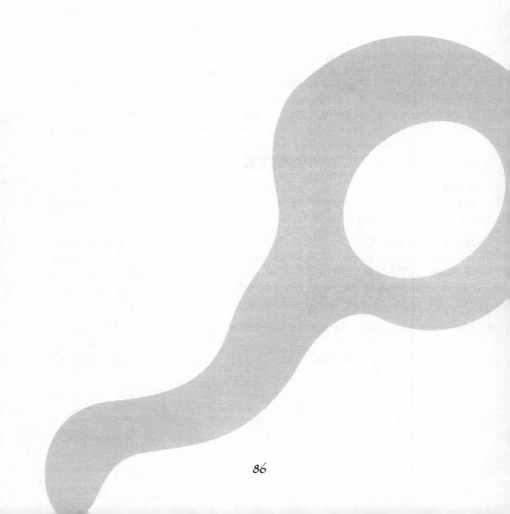

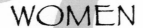

WOMEN

Women have spent much of history as little more than property of their husbands. Their role, throughout most of civilization's cultures, has been as their mate's helpers, usually having no real identity of their own:

It was not until late in the history of the Roman Empire that women had individual names. If the husband's last name was Claudius, she was Claudia, and likewise with other family names. If there was more than one woman in the family, she was called either "the elder" or "the younger."

The sons in the Fanti tribe inherited the wives of their fathers upon the father's death. All his father's wives were then his, except for his biological mother.

In parts of India, a man's wife could be taken as security. A man owing a debt to another could have his wife taken from him until the debt was paid.

The creditor had all the rights to the woman that the husband had. Children born out of the union between the creditor and the debtor's wife were split between the two men.

That women have been treated as merchandise is obvious. However, this attitude is commonly associated only with primitive or Eastern cultures:

It was not uncommon for women to be bought and sold through newspaper advertisements in 18th-century Ireland. The standard offer to sell a woman: "A bargain to be sold."

The selling of wives occurred as recently as the 18th century in Europe. Though the practice was frowned upon, it was tolerated. There is record of a Scotsman who sold his wife by weight—at two pence per pound.

In some periods, the disgust toward a woman who had been enjoyed by another man was so extreme as to justify getting rid of her, whether she be married or not. Such has been the reaction to a woman who had been sexually violated:

Adam of Bremen, writing in the last half of the 11th century, made it law that the Danish woman who had been raped should be sold into slavery.

The 4000-year-old Babylonian Code of Hammurabi assigned the same punishment to the victim as to the offender of rape. Both the man and his victim had their hands and feet tied and were thrown into the Euphrates or Tigris Rivers.

In rare instances, women have been known to rape:

The women of the Kogi tribe in Colombia were in the habit of ambushing men and raping them.

Prices have long been attached to women:

In Papua New Guinea, men purchased their wives by paying a dowry. An unmarried woman cost cash, one bird and five pigs. A previously married woman, either divoced or widowed, cost about one-tenth of the cash for a new bride, a bird and two pigs. The woman who had been married twice had no dowry at all.

On the island of Unamarck, women were used as money. All items that had trading value were priced by their cost in women.

In Fiji, women were often used to buy things. At one point, the value of one woman was equal, for trading purposes, to that of a pig.

Many different cultures treated women as either annoying, boldly deceitful or extremely dangerous:

In the Chinese manuscript *Tso-chuan*, written about 635 B.C., it was said of females: "The te (bewitching power) of a girl is without limits, the resentment of a married woman is without end."

The English woman during the Renaissance was not well respected in matters of honesty. A certain Father Gury found difficulty in hearing women's confessions, because "women are habitually inclined to lie."

Even Confucius, the sage of ancient China, was mystified by the nature of women. He considered them "difficult to deal with. If you are friendly with them, they get out of hand, and if you keep your distance, they resent it."

An Arab saying concerning the nature of women: "Women are made of nectar and poison."

The Medieval Arab writer Ghazali was critical of "troublesome" women: "It is a fact that all trials, misfortunes, and woes which befall men, come from women."

An old Arab saying claimed that the "straightest woman is as twisted as a sickle."

The Indian laws of Manu proclaimed that "the cause of dishonor is woman; the cause of hostility is woman; the cause of worldly things is woman; therefore woman should be shunned."

At times, the value placed on women was very low:

When Europeans appeared in New Caledonia, they introduced the flint-lock musket. The chief of one of the tribes, in testing this new piece of equipment, set his wives up in a row. He then began shooting them as if in a shooting gallery.

A New Caledonian native man asked the missionary of the area to baptize him into the Catholic faith. The clergyman told him that since he was living with a woman in sin, he could not be baptized. The next day, the man returned to the missionary. The problem was solved, he said; he was no longer living in sin. He could now be baptized. He had killed his wife and eaten her.

In many cultures, private passion was paired with public indifference:

Chinese Confucianists held the belief that outside of the bedchamber, the husband should show little interest in his wife.

♀

The church alternately characterized the woman as a slave of her sexual impulses, and as the victim of men's sexual desires. She has been cast as wanton, sexually depraved, and a temptress of lust. Just as often, she has been presented as the unwilling object of sex, the pure, innocent, unwilling party:

The medieval church viewed woman as sexually evil. St. Chrysostom (347–407) was quoted by the holy men of that time as saying that females were "a necessary evil, a natural temptation, a desirable calamity, a domestic peril, a deadly fascination, and a painted ill."

♀

Throughout the course of history, the male has been known as having a very healthy sexual appetite. This has not been the case with women. The belief in their desire, or lack of desire, has fluctuated. The Victorian view, for instance, of a woman without any sexual appetite is very different from the opinion of those of older societies:

The Bible had this to say of the sexual desires of women: "Three things are insatiable...hell, the mouth of the vulva, and the earth."

♀

The belief in woman's craving for sexual pleasure has resulted in severe injustice:

The Talmud, the ancient Jewish scripture, did not truly believe in women's fear or disgust of rape. Rape was not considered a serious crime. It was believed that often the nature of woman might overcome the initial horror of the act and realize "an inward instinctual consent."

♀

The Arabs believed that after sex with a woman, a man must thoroughly wash his whole body. A common saying was, "Wash thoroughly after lying with a woman, or no horse worth its salt will permit you to mount it."

Iraqi women were obliged to wash themselves thoroughly immediately after intercourse. They were not allowed to leave the room until they had done this. If a woman had been discovered to have broken this rule, she was whipped.

♀

The Christian Church did not consider women's bodies in any more flattering light:

St. Augustine (A.D. 354–430) proclaimed, "The body of a man is superior to that of a woman as the soul is to the body."

Men of science often thought no differently:

Aristotle (384–322 B.C.), philosopher: "Just as it sometimes happens that deformed offspring are produced by deformed parents, and sometimes not, so the offspring produced by a female are sometimes female, sometimes not, but male. The reason is that the female is as it were a deformed male...we should look upon the female state as being...a deformity."

A certain few societies have treated women as equals:

On long hunting trips, it was standard practice for the men of some American Indian tribes to hire a girl to accompany them. The girl did all the things the male did: hunting, fishing and curing the meat. She also provided sexual companionship. She was given a fair share of the goods, and the arrangement was usually ended upon the return to the village. Nothing more was expected from either party.

Hippocrates, Greek physician and teacher of medicine (460–377 B.C.), spoke of the existence of a Scythian people living near the Sea of Azor. They were called Sauromatrians. The women rode horseback, fought in wars while they were virgins and did not marry until they had skinned three enemies.

Once married, these women stopped riding and ceased to be part of the army unless the nation was in great danger. These women were all missing the right breast, which was destroyed in childhood. This was done by the girls' mothers. It was believed that the breast sapped the strength of the arm and shoulder of that side of the body, so it was destroyed to make the women more powerful.

In some other societies, women held higher status than men:

In ancient Arabia, it was the women who possessed the majority of the wealth. Very often they owned large flocks of sheep and herds of cattle. The husband was, subsequently, merely the herdsman for her property. A common declaration of divorce was, "I will no longer drive your flocks to the pasture."

Women's main function in history has been that of childbearer. At times it has seemed to be her only function:

Plutarch was a Greek essayist and biographer (A.D. 50–120). He described, in a work called *Lycurgus*, the marital habits of Spartan husbands and wives: Spartan marriages were curiously lacking in love and affection. Unlike the Greeks, Spartans married full-grown women.

A Spartan kidnapped the woman he desired, and she was placed in the care of a femal attendant, Her hair was cut short, and she was dressed in a male's tunic and sandals. She was laid on a mattress of straw, in the darkness.

The groom had dinner, as always, with his friends, in the dormitory (nearly all Spartans were soldiers). Then, taking care not to be discovered, he escaped the company of his friends to go to his bride. He removed her belt and carried her to bed. After having sex and not much else, he hurried back to the dormitory.

He followed this schedule every day, socializing with his male friends all day and night, and slipping away in secret to meet his wife for a quick bout of sex. These proceedings lasted so long that often a husband had several children by the woman whose face he'd never seen in the light of day.

While sex has usually been a private matter, childbirth often wasn't:

In Kamchatka, women gave birth in public, in the middle of the village.

A small amount of empathy has been shown the woman who gave birth:

The Greek historian Siculus noted an ancient Greek custom on the island of Corsica. After the delivery of a new child, a Corsican father would take to his bed. There he would rest, as if it were he who had suffered the labor his wife had gone through.

Plutarch saw a similar custom on the island of Cyprus. In this case, when the woman was taken to bed to deliver, the husband did the same. He would cry and shake along with his wife, she giving birth, he going through the motions.

Natives of Guiana were observed by the adventurer Brett. Brett saw the new father of a child lay in his hammock for several days, pretending to be ill. He lay stark naked in an immodest position, accepting the concern and good wishes of the female neighbors. The new mother, by this time, was already back to her normal duties, in addition to caring for the baby. By this time she was generally ignored.

In contrast to her great value as a childbearer, a woman was restricted by many cultures because of her capacity to bear children. Menstruation made the woman an object of disgust, and often she was shunned because of her menstrual condition:

Starting with the Chinese Chou dynasty (1500–771 B.C.), it was the practice of women who had their monthly flow to put a red spot on their foreheads to announce the fact that they were having their period, and impure.

In some parts of India, a woman who was having her period advertised her condition by wearing a small scarf around her neck, onto which was smeared some of her menstrual blood.

In ancient China, women in the province of Tsinhai were very careful at the time of their period. To make sure that no menstrual blood fell on the ground, they tied their clothes to their ankles. It was believed that should a drop of blood fall to the earth, the earth spirit would be disgusted and sentence the girl to hell.

Among the North Queensland Australian aborigines, a girl who had her first period was taken from the village and buried up to her waist in the ground. Then a circle of brushwood was built around her to keep her out of sight. Not only was nobody allowed to touch her she was not even allowed to touch herself. Her mother fed her and provided her with a stick in case she needed to scratch herself.

In West Africa, in the Assini region, women were not allowed to cross the river either by themselves or by canoe during their period. Should they have tried to do this, it would have provoked the anger of the gods.

Ancient Persians severely limited the activities of a woman having her period. She could not speak to men or look into the "sacred fire." Neither was she allowed to look at the sun or sit in the water at the time of menstruation.

Angolan women having their periods were obligated to hide themselves away for a period of six days, roughly the length of their periods. To avoid disaster, they were warnted not to touch or even look at cow dung.

Dr. Bertherand related that in the Arab world, the repulsion to a woman having her period was extreme. At the time of his observance in the 19th century, and likely for many, many years before, the man who was familiar with his wife during her period was considered lowly. In fact, "the judicial testimony of a man who has cohabitated with his wife during her menstrual period will be unacceptable."

Women have had to show great courage in the job of maternity:

South American mothers had to be very restrained in childbirth; should they have moaned or groaned, the newborn child was killed.

The menstrual flow has had its positive side:

The woman of the Beaver Indian tribe allowed herself 10 days to have and recover from her period. At this time she was usually in bad temper and refused any sexual advances her husband made. Once the husband understood this, it allowed her more time to be with her lovers.

The timing of the woman's period could be hazardous:

In some parts of India, if a woman was having her period at the same time as the death of her husband, she was burned alive.

The mystery of the female body and the secret of menstruation has also caused cultures to believe in its magical and healing powers:

The East African Warundi girl who had her period was considered diseased and could not take part in everyday life for this period of time. However, she was taken once into the hut to "bless" everything inside with her touch.

Cappadocian women, said Pliny (Italian scholar, A.D. 23–79), were very useful to their farming husbands. Menstruating women were carried through the fields to save the crops from worms and insects.

The ancient Greeks believed that the woman who had her period had great power. Pliny noted: "Hailstorms, they say, whirlwinds and lightnings, even, will be scared away by a woman uncovering her body while her monthly courses are upon her. At any other time, also, if a woman strips herself naked while she is menstruating, and walks round a field of wheat, the caterpillars, worms, beetles, and other vermin will fall from off the ears of corn."

The men of the Pacific Ainu tribe considered menstrual blood a good-luck charm, and would beg a woman to get part of the cloth she used between her legs.

In central Australia, a seriously ill or dying man was often treated with blood taken from a cut made in the vaginal lips of a woman.

The mystery of women's bodies has caused much trouble:

In Ireland, it was believed that a woman's menopause provoked common and permanent madness in her. They did not realize that it was only the temporary menopause itself that was the trouble. To guard against going mad during menopause, many women completely withdrew from everyday life once they reached their 40s.

Women's anatomy has long been one of mankind's greatest curiosities:

Ancient Mesopotamian medical men believed it was possible to tell the sex of a child before it was born. They believed the child was female if the mother's forehead was clear-skinned. If she developed freckles on her forehead, they predicted the birth of a boy.

The ancient Egyptians believed that should expectant mothers acquire a taste for sour things, the embryo would lay farther to the left of the womb, and be a boy. If the mothers were fond of sweet things, having the embryo shift to the right, the mother could be sure the baby was a girl.

In the 19th century, it was believed that the position of the woman during and following intercourse decided the sex of her child. A boy was the result of his mother lying on her right side while having sex, and lying on that side afterward. A daughter was produced from the mother's position being on the left.

A certain Dr. Guillon, in 1877, put forward a theory that he could determine the sex of a child by the mother's excrement. A male would be born to a woman with "dense, reddish, rounded, fatty" stool. A girl was to be expected if the feces were pale and flat.

Aretaeus of Cappadocia, who lived in the time of ancient Greek influence, was a writer who believed that the uterus was like a wandering animal. This was a common belief of the time. He was of the opinion that the uterus lay in the abdomen of the woman but could also move to either side of the woman's body.

The Greek teacher and philosopher Aristotle (384–322 B.C.) discussed the womb in his work *Timaeus*. He believed that if a woman had a long period of fertility without conceiving, the womb became irritated and dissatisfied. It wandered the body, choking and stifling the woman's breathing. It complained bitterly by initiating any number of sicknesses.

Galen was a Greco-Roman physician who lived from A.D. 129 to 199. He believed that the womb was happy only when being exercised. Withholding the liquid of the womb by not experiencing orgasm, he believed, caused a poisoning of the blood, cooling of the body and nervous irritation. Thus, to stay healthy, Galen prescribed regular intercourse. If this was not possible, Galen recommended periodic masturbation.

At the time of the Plague, between 1347 and 1350, it was advised that sexual contact with women be avoided. Sleeping with a woman, or even coming in contact with her bed, supposedly increased the threat of contracting the Black Death.

The medieval French friar Luis de Leon noted, "Nature made women slow in movement so that they might be easy on their clothes."

Fertility ceremonies have been a staple of sexual rites—with women playing a very active part:

Diodorus, who visited ancient Egypt from 60 to 57 B.C., witnessed an Egyptian fertility rite. It involved installing a bull in the sanctuary of Hephaestus at Memphis. This sacred Apis bull was put on a barge in a luxurious compartment and taken to the sanctuary down the waterway. To stimulate the god's virility, the women lifted their dresses and exposed their genitals to the bull. This lasted 40 days; men were not allowed to view the bull. Thereafter, women were forbidden to see the Apis bull.

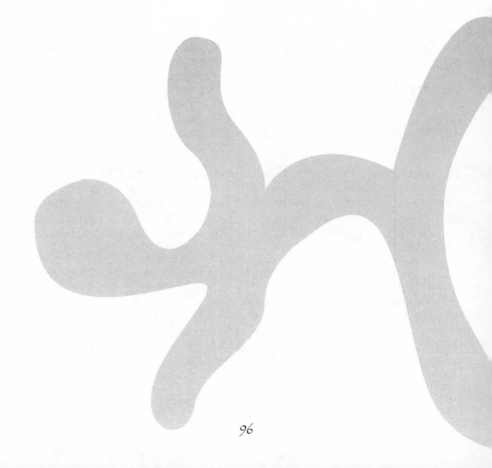

PUBERTY

Puberty rites often reflected the "death" of a child and its rebirth as an adult:

Among Amazonian tribes such as the Mandrucus, the dead were sewed up in a cloth bag. Similarly, they laid a girl who had reached womanhood into a cloth hammock, and sewed it up so that the only opening was a small hole for breathing. Then a low fire was built underneath the sack, and the girl was left hanging over the fire for several days.

Among primitive tribes, the boy who has attained manhood and the right to sexual activity has undergone much pain. This pain has been seen as necessary to show his courage and manliness:

In Guiana, Macusi boys entering into manhood were tested for their bravery. They were soundly flogged and prodded with wild boar tusks. Then they were taken to a hammock and sewed into it with hundreds of stinging bugs. He was obligated to say nothing while undergoing this test. If he yelled or cried out, he was not allowed to ever marry.

In southern Australia, there was practiced a particularly painful puberty rite. When a boy reached the age of manhood, he was christened with tree boughs. Then he was sprinkled with the blood of a warrior. The young man was then buried in the earth and sprinkled with dust. After being covered to the neck, he was then pulled out by his ears.

The South American Mura puberty initiation was a dangerous affair. The boys were obligated to drink a very large amount of liquor. Then the women of the village gave the boys enemas. This forced their bellies to swell to large proportions and put their intestines under great pressure. In this condition, the boys performed vigorous exercises, the result sometimes being that an unfortunate boy's belly exploded.

While the boy or girl undergoing the initiation has usually been the object of abuse, in some societies his or her failures could have larger consequences:

The Naivasha Masai boys were not allowed to cry out while undergoing his initiation. If he did so, he was considered a coward and expelled from the tribe. His family had to pay a fine, and each member of his family was soundly beaten.

Puberty rites have typically focused on the genitals, the capacity and responsibility to procreate being a gift of maturity:

A boy of the African Chaggas could not have sex until he had gone through the initiation into manhood. If he was caught having sex, he was taken to the center of the village and laid on his partner, and both were staked to the ground in this position.

The ancient Greek boy who reached maturity was now obligated to show a sense of modesty toward his penis. This was accomplished by having the foreskin drawn over the glans and securely tied. Apparently this was done to protect the boy's penises during gymnastics. It must also have discouraged sexual excitement, as an erection would have caused a lot of pain.

The Punjabi Pathans circumcised their boys as part of their puberty rites. The foreskin was then buried in the ground, usually in a damp part of the house, such as the spot where the water jars were kept. The foreskin would then grow and his manhood would be increased.

Bala boys in the Congo, between the ages of 7 and 12, were obligated to submit to the puberty rite of circumcision. Once the boy's foreskin was removed, a banana leaf was wrapped around it.

It was then placed on a termite hill to be consumed by the insects. This was vital; if the foreskin was not devoured, it was believed the boy would not grow up to be potent. The patient's wound was cleaned, and the boy stood in front of a fire for one day and the following night, with the penis catching the smoke of the fire. Until the boy's surgery had healed, his mother and father were not allowed to have intercourse.

The Chuka and Amwimbe practiced circumcision. Only part of the foreskin was removed. After this portion of the foreskin was cut off, making a hole in the foreskin, the boy's glans, or head of the penis, was pushed through this hole.

The Samoan boy between the ages of 10 and 12 went through puberty ceremonies that included being tossed in the air, being beaten by men of the tribe and having his scalp carved. The boy's younger brother was also involved in the puberty rite. When the older brother was circumcised, the foreskin was given to the younger brother. This foreskin, to ensure strength and vitality, was eaten by the younger boy.

Tahitian boys aged 11 to 15 submitted themselves to a circumcision ceremony to achieve manhood. The boys lined up and, one by one, walked a distance to the circumciser. Each squatted down, and his penis was placed on a halved coconut shell. His foreskin was tightly pulled over the head of his penis and onto the shell. The foreskin was cut on the shell while an assistant restrained the boy by holding on to his ears.

The initiation ceremony for the Nandi was held for groups of boys every four years. The boy borrowed all kinds of jewelry and clothing from the girls. He decorated himself with flowers as well. The elder of the village asked the group of boys if they had experienced intercourse with a circumcised (and therefore married) woman. Any boy asked this was usually absolutely honest in his response, even though a yes meant a severe beating for the woman whose name he provided. The boy's head was painted white, and he was brought to the circumciser. His foreskin was pulled, and a hot iron run around the skin. Fat was applied to the wound and in a matter of days the foreskin whithered and fell off. The boy did not yell; if he did so, he was run through with a spear.

The Sebeyi boy underwent the following circumcision rite: The boy held a long stick above his head. He was covered with bull's intestines. As he stood, two men circumcised him. He could not alter his rigid position. Following the circumcision, the boy jumped up and down, holding the bull's stomach in his hands. He kept jumping up and down until an elder forced him to sit down. As the villagers gathered around, the boy tossed his head from side to side. His mother, spitting at intervals, brought him milk. But she could not approach him directly—she had to weave a path toward him. Once he got the milk from her, he drank it, taking care not to spill any. If he spilled it on his penis, it was believed that it would fall off. Afterward, he had to spit three times on everything he touched. His mother could not see him while he was healing. If by accident she saw him, she threw her skirt over her head and ran away.

The Kenyan Kipsigis held initiation rites for boys 14 to 18. The group of initiates was organized under the leadership of an elder. He acted as foreman to the boys in the construction of a ceremonial hut. Its main feature was a hallway constructed from sticks. On these sticks were stinging nettles. At the end of the passageway was constructed a completely dark room.

When finished, each young man stood in front of his parents' hut, dressed in his best finery. The women of the village, looking their best, danced and sang for them. In the evening, the warriors danced, and all wives had intercourse with whomever they pleased.

The morning after the dance and mate-swapping, the boys went to the ceremonial hut. Each boy was obligated to pass through the hallway of stinging nettles four times.

Then he was taken to the dark room, and sat down next to a heap of monkey skins. A confessor told the boy that he must truthfully confess, or the beast under the monkey skins, Arap Mogoss, would visit the youth in the night and kill him. It was explained that the animal has a huge penis, which he would use on the boy if he lied.

The boy was then asked about his sex life, and more specifically, if he had experienced intercourse. To scare the boy into telling the truth, the monkey skins started to move, and Mogoss began to make low, threatening "mooing" sounds.

If he still denied having had intercourse, another voice, sounding somewhat like a woman, accused the boy of having slept with her, giving all the details of the supposed lovemaking session. At the same time there was a wet, sucking sound coming out from the skins. A thick stick was moved in and out of a small waterhole. It was the simulated sound of a penis in a vagina.

If the boy insisted on his innocence, the confessor was satisfied and the boy was set free. Later, he was circumcised.

Torres Straits natives believed that the onset of a girl's period was the result of the moon having had sex with her.

When Tahitian girls started menstruating, this occasion was received with joy. Tahitians believed that if girls did not menstruate at the proper time, the blood would go to their heads and kill them.

The girl who reached puberty was considered mature, but to have the capacity of a woman, she had to undergo physical tests:

The Tlinkit girl's first menstruation was physically demanding. On evidence of her period, she was taken to a secluded hut. There she was under strict orders not to lie down. She was provided with logs to lean on as she slept sitting up. Charcoal was smeared onto her face, and her head was wrapped in a woven mat. This was done to keep her from being exposed to the light of day. Her helplessness was so complete that she was not allowed to chew her own food. This was done for her by one of her family.

The Ticuna girl, upon menstruating, was confined to a completely closed off hut. Then she was beaten and had every hair on her head pulled out.

The African girl in Glenel, Victoria, was required to have a large vagina to accommodate intercourse. If she was examined and found not to have a sufficiently large vagina, it was enlarged (or believed to be enlarged) by inserting the head of a snake.

The snake, or serpent, has been a common symbol among many cultures:

In Bolivia, when a Chiriguano girl experienced her first menstruation, the elder woman took up sticks and searched for the snake which had bitten the girl to cause her period.

The time of puberty was one of great expectation for the girl. She was usually elevated in status after passing through girlhood because of her new capacity as a wife and mother. For the girls in some tribes, they were nonpersons until they had the ability to reproduce:

Among the Chukchee tribe of Paleo-Siberia, there was no definite word to describe a girl. Instead, she was referred to as *yep ayaakelen*, meaning "not yet put in use."

The central Australian Aranda girl was married to several men when she reached puberty. Her husbands were much older than she was. This marriage did not make them wives, however; it made them, technically, mothers-in-law, because their husbands, by marrying the girls, were entitled to marry their daughters.

The young woman was sometimes tested for her sexual purity:

Girls in Iceland who exhibited ticklishness as a test of their purity were treated with scorn. Their ticklishness was thought to be a sign that they had lost their virginity.

In some cultures, the girl who reached the age of fertility was considered valuable enough to need protective magic charms, and in one case in particular, a sort of guardian angel:

In some parts of Africa, the cow was considered holy. It was not sold or loaned out. It was a "sister" to the family's daughter, and by this sisterhood conferred its power, health and fertility to the girl. The girl's father ripped a few hairs out of his most attractive cow's vulva. The girl's mother braided these hairs and hung this strange necklace around her daughter's neck.

The magic of the changes of puberty has been a source of fear as well as reverence:

Among the Carrier Indians of British Columbia, Canada, there was a curious practice. Young native girls who began menstruating were banished from the village. With the onset of their first period, they were sent into the wilderness for three or four years. It was considered dangerous for anyone to see them while they were banished. They were said to taint any paths that they crossed while separated from the tribe.

The Thonga girls of Southwest Africa, at the age of puberty, were kept away from the rest of the tribe. They wore a dirty, greasy veil, and every morning bathed. While they went to the bath, and while bathing, the older girls and women sang obscene songs. They also beat any men they came upon with sticks. Any man found near their camp was seized and asked about the female circumcision ceremony—including obscene words and descriptions. If he didn't or couldn't answer these deliberately very sexual questions, he was beaten.

Puberty has signified the time when the new adult was freed from the protective eye of the parents:

The Yukaghirs of Paleo-Siberia allowed the pubescent girl her privacy. When she had her first period, she set up a separate tent for herself away from the family. She retreated to this tent at night only, so that she could receive her lovers without any obstacles.

Aboriginal tribes have treated the emergence of manhood and woman-hood with an openness and frankness alien to more complex societies:

The East African Kikuyu girl underwent a long puberty ceremony. Shortly after her pubic hair made its appearance, at about 12 years of age, she borrowed clothes and ornaments from her male relatives. In the evening she was taken by a female elder of the village. She spread her legs and the woman examined her to see if she was still a virgin. If she was, all the women in the village kissed her, and her father set a feast for the village. Stinging nettles were placed on her clitoris, and she went the whole night with these nettles attached. This made the clitoris swell fiercely. The next day the female elder applied a hot coal to the girl's clitoris. The woman raised a cry, likely to muffle the girl's cry. If her father heard her cry, he had the right to run a spear through her. She went off to live by herself for four months and was not allowed to be seen by a man. If she was, she starved herself to death, unless she could rub a palmful of the man's spit on her forehead.

The Kenyan Nandi tribe practiced group female circumcision. At the age of 10, the clitoris and lips of the vagina were removed. Before this surgery, the girls were obligated to sleep with boys in a hut specifically designed for this function. If they refused, they were beaten. It was understood that no sexual activity was allowed, and the following morning they were examined to determine if they had kept their virginity. If they had, they were rewarded with cattle. If they did not show the physical signs of sexual innocence, they were speared to death.

Sexual initiation has been a feature of puberty rites:

At the age of puberty, Australian aborigine girls were circumcised with a stone knife by the boys in their tribe. The removal of the clitoris meant that the girl was now pure and sexually desirable. After this operation was performed, the boys of the tribe had group sex with her.

When a Kaffir girl reached puberty, it was celebrated by a festival. At this festival the girl was honored, and it was announced that she was ready to lay with any and all who came to her.

When a young Japanese girl in the Heian age had experienced her first period, a ceremony was held. The boys of the village were lined up in two rows, facing each other. The new woman had a silk flag tucked into her sash. As she ran down the corridor between the two lines of boys, they attempted to yank the silk flag off her sash. The boy who got the flag took the girl home and took her virginity.

Among some tribes in the Cameroons, the boy's initiation took as long as six months. For this time, they lived in the forest away from the village, with the "priests" of the tribe. When the initiation was over, a spear was thrust out of each of the young men's huts. They then appeared publicly for the first time with tattooed faces.

The newly initiated Cameroon girls did the same thing. The boys lined up facing the line of the girls. They danced, then threw off their banana-girdles and had sex.

Many of the puberty initiations have been very practical affairs:

Among Peruvian and Amazon basin tribes, the initiate girl was made drunk. She was circumcised, and a clay penis of the same size as her fiance's penis was introduced into her vagina. Now a true woman, she could be married.

In central Africa, in Azimbaland, the initiation ceremony for a girl experiencing her first period dealt with her sexual education. To ready her for sexual intercourse, the girl was often subjected to surgery of a sort. A corn cob, or perhaps a horn, was tied to a girdle of bark and inserted into the girl's vagina. This was done to make her vagina more accommodating to intercourse. She was then taught the various love-making positions. Her period having passed, the girdle was removed, and a morning dance, open only to the females of the village, was held. The girl was led from her mother's hut and sat down, the other village women standing in a circle around her. Several songs referring to the girl's genitals were sung. Then she was stripped bare and made to go through the motions of intercourse. If she did not do this to satisfaction, the other women corrected her, taking her place and acting out the proper method.

In many cultures, sexual initiation has typically been left to fumbling novices of the same tender age. But there are traditions by which the older tutor introduced the virgin to pleasures of the flesh:

Marquesan boys were initiated into the sexual act at the age of 12 or 13—a little later than their sisters. The boy's first sexual experience was usually with an older woman whose husband was away from the village.

In New Hebrides, all young men who had been circumcised, lived in Imeium ("youth's house"). While there they were visited at certain times of the year by an Iowhanan girl from another village. This Iowhanan was well dressed and painted differently from other girls. She also wore her skirt shorter. She gave newly circumcised males a practical course in sex while she lived in the Imeium, and when all were educated, returned to her village, honor intact. No male was ever allowed to be married without having been initiated by the Iowhanan girl.

SELECTING A MATE

In Persia a girl could marry only with the approval of her parents. But a young man who did not want to risk rejection by parents, and who wanted to make sure that he got his love before all others, could avoid this procedure.

If he seized the girl, cut off a length of her hair, tore her veil away and threw a sheet over her, announcing her as his wife, he was formally engaged.

That men show absolute proof of their masculinity has been a common requisite for both primitive and "cultured" peoples:

In the age of chivalry in France, a knight, if he did not have a reputation for bravery already, had to prove his worthiness to the lady from whom he wanted attentions. This was not his choice; he did not prove his value to impress her. She absolutely demanded it. The common statement on the part of the woman was: "I care only that your sword be sharp. It is necessary that for your love of me you should do deeds of chivalry."

The natives of Jebel Nyima in Nubia often entertained guests with the utmost courtesy and in the most generous fashion. However, after the guest left the household, the host often slit the guest's throat. This was necessary for the host to be able to marry, as he was not eligible to take a bride until he had committed a murder.

Standards for measuring eligibility of a mate have been very different throughout the world:

The Moravians had a very systematic way of pairing off. A man notified his priest of his desire to take a wife. The priest advised a superintendent of young women, who notified the priest of the next eligible girl on her list. The two singles met for an hour, and if both were agreeable, married the following day. If there was no match, the girl's name was put at the bottom of the eligibility list, and the man was obligated to stay single forever—unless he, or the girl, decided on second thought to marry each other anyway.

In some parts of Brazil, men had very specific requirements for their wives. The most prized bride was the girl who was a good gardener and made good beer.

The Russians of the 15th century never exhibited their daughters, and a marriage was made without either party having seen the other. Later, under Peter the Great, the couple were still engaged through their parents, without their consent. However, if the man and woman did not know each other, the families arranged to conveniently meet by "accident." The young man's father then invited the bride's father to meet again, both families being present, to formalize the arrangement.

The Central Asian Kirghis were not interested in the good-looking and young women, considering them useless. The men chose older, faded women whom they knew to be skilled and hard workers.

In the age of chivalry in England, jousting tournaments were frequently held as occasions to find a girl a husband. Such was the case when William Peverel disposed of his niece, Melette, as the prize of the winner of the tournament. This was the only way in which the girl had agreed to be married.

In Gambia, a man had several wives, with one being more privileged than the others. This wife was called the chief wife. This favored wife was not the prettiest, or the youngest, or the most sexually satisfying wife. The qualification as a man's favorite was her talent as a good business manager.

The men of many parts of Africa, including the Baholoholo, the Nandi, the Bandiagoro and the Homlosi, disliked the idea of marrying virgins. In fact, the most desirable women, to these men, were those who had already had a child, for good reason: She had already proved her reproductive worth.

Among most Polynesian tribes, one of the best qualifications for a wife to have was a good tattoo. A man serious about marrying demanded to check his prospective bride's tattoo, to ensure that she was "protected" from misfortune. This was common policy, so the unmarried women very willingly allowed the men to examine the tattoos on their vulvae.

Among some cultures, possible mates were clearly defined:

The Hindus, ever interested in the science of sex, labeled men and women into different types. There were four types of women:

- Pudminee, the Lotus Woman. The perfect woman. She was well mannered and delicately built.

- Chitrinee, the Art Woman. She was more worldly than the Pudminee, and almost as delicately proportioned.

- Sunkhinee, the Shell Woman. The common sort of woman. Hard working and of good breeding stock, she is a little heavier-set than either the Pudminee or Chitrinee.

- Hustinee, the Elephant Woman. The least desirable sort of woman. Somewhat lazier and heavy-built. Coarse and sexually insatiable.

Hindu males were of four types, according to the Indian sexologists:

- Shushah, the Hare Man. The perfect male, lean and strong, with a small, lean penis.

- Mrigah, the Buck Man. The ideal warrior. Quick and graceful, his penis is longer and thicker than the Shushah's.

- Vrishubha, the Bull Man. Tough and muscular. Penis is of above average length.

- Ushvah, the Stallion Man. Lazy and witless, he is good only for procreation. Is grotesquely overendowed.

In some places, the method of choosing a mate was less particular:

The Dinka woman's only status was in the value of her marriage dowry. Because of this, these women preferred to marry a man they did not like who offered a larger dowry, than marry the man of their choice who could provide only a smaller dowry.

Albanian girls looking for husbands advertised their availability, as well as the reward for their hand in marriage. The single girls wore red caps with rows of coins attached, like fish scales, to advertise the good fortune of a match with them.

In certain areas of Mexico, a man wishing to marry went to a temple and advised the priest of this. In front of the rest of the church, some of his hair was cut off, and he proclaimed his readiness and willingness to take a wife. As he left the temple, he was required to marry the first single girl he came upon.

In some parts of Central Africa, it was believed that a girl with high, firm breasts was infertile. For this reason, the only requirement women had to have was flabby, long and drooping breasts.

In Somali, the man looking for a wife gathered together all the single women. They lined up in a row, and he stepped behind the lineup, choosing as his wife the girl with the biggest buttocks.

The Persians designated men as being of three types: the proper man, the half-man and the hupal-hupla:

- The proper man never went out without his wife's permission and was always obedient. The proper man always provided for the woman whatever she desired.

- The half-man was a poor provider, and the woman who married this man had to work herself. Because of this, she was entitled to argue with him, even merely to show her general dissatisfaction with him.

- The hupal-hupla man was considered the most materially miserable of men. This man was not entitled to question his wife about her absences, no matter how lengthy. He could not enter his own house when the door was shut, but was obligated to stay away until the door was opened. He could not ask what his wife was doing in the company of a stranger, or what the stranger's relationship with her was. If he did any of this, she was entitled to divorce him at once.

The Guana girl chose the eligibility of the man who wanted her by going to his parents. She very specifically asked what she was obligated to do, and how much. She asked if she was required to help build the hut, collect firewood, tend to the garden, make blankets and cook, and to what degree. As well, she asked if he was to have any other wives, and how often she was required to sleep with him. It was only after carefully outlining these points that she decided whether or not to stay with him.

One of the most common features of mate selection throughout the world has been the emphasis placed on wealth:

The Brazilian Carajas society favored older men. The older and subsequently usually wealthier men monopolized the women. The younger Carajas men, consequently, were forced to take older women as temporary wives until they could earn their fortune and be able to get their choice of wives.

In Russia, St. Petersburg had a garden called Bride's Fair. A man looking for a wife frequented this garden. Eligible women were seen in their finest, including lace, jewels, silver teaspoons, fancy plates and whatever other household treasures they could offer.

The Hill Damaras people exchanged dowries, but for the most part it was more of symbolic value than anything else. A perfectly acceptable bride's dowry could be a handful of onions and some mice.

The Fan tribe of Africa valued women highly, and their dowries were high. The father, demanding his due, lavished praise on his daughter in selling her to the prospective husband. The groom-to-be, however, insulted and ridiculed her, hoping to reduce her dowry price. Caught between the two, the girl took it all in stride.

The Kaffir girl adorned herself in a most flattering way, then proceeded to the groom's hut. There, the men of the village were gathered. She knelt down, took her clothes off and called attention to her best qualities. She then sat humbly and quietly as the men argued the virtues and shortcomings of her body. They discussed any and all of her most private parts with enthusiasm or disdain. Then the women of the village poked and prodded her body, examining her further. It was only then that the price of her dowry was discussed.

While the idea of purchasing a mate, whether through dowry, prearranged matches or simple purchase, seems uncivilized, this practice has occurred until relatively recent times:

As late as the 19th century, women were being bought and sold on a regular and organized basis. In England, many husbands went to the market to sell their wives. A man usually threw a rope around his wife's neck, led her to the market and tied her to a post. Side by side with the other commodities, such as cattle, she was sold to the highest bidder.

The buyer, for his part, was acknowledged as the lawful mate of the purchased woman, and her children were regarded as his own. It was common that a trip to the market was followed by a trip to the church to formalize the union.

While the sale of women has been well documented, there are rarer but nonetheless existent cases of men being sold by their wives:

Up to the 19th century, English husbands were sold by their wives. While women were sold at what seems a very small price, often as little as one guinea, husbands generally went even more cheaply.

Buying the companionship of women is universal in the world. However, in some rare instances, men could be "bought":

The Sumatran Alfur girl who could not readily find a husband could still often enjoy male companionship. Her father often paid young men to court her until the right husband showed up.

Selecting a mate has usually involved some form of exchange of affection or show of love by test of courage. But there have been other ways to win a woman:

Aetans of the Philippine Islands had a very modest way of choosing a mate. The young man inquired a girl's parents as to their daughter. They sent her into the forest before dawn. The boy was required to leave his hut an hour later. If he could not find the girl and bring her back before sunset, he was refused any further chance to marry her.

The Maori man of New Zealand could have many wives. Young or old, pretty or plain, they all shared the same status, with one exception: The first wife to give birth to a son became the favored wife.

The large majority of cultures had dictated the eligibility of a mate by strict kinship qualifications. In most cases, the object has been to have marriages to nonrelatives, to enlarge the clan. But there have been exceptions:

The Arab, according to Mohammed, was to have one wife, ideally. This woman was usually his first cousin. If she preferred another man, she was required to get her male cousin's permission, even if he already had another wife.

Should a South African of the Herero tribe become attached to a girl who was her family's younger sister, he had a special obligation. The man could not marry the younger sister without marrying the older one as well.

Among some of the Omaha and California Indians, it was common for a man to take as his bride his niece or an aunt.

The people of the New Guinea Mundugumor tribe practiced a sometimes complicated form of mating. The boys of the tribe traded their sisters for their wives. This could be complicated if, for instance, a young boy had a sister much older than himself. No matter how young the boy, it was absolutely necessary that a wife be found for the boy before the sister was claimed. His "wife," then, could either be several years older than him, or a mere baby.

In a large number of the world's families, the parents have had an absolute right to choose a husband or wife:

In Africa, when a young Basuto man's parents saw him leading the cows out of the pen, they understood his message, and immediately set to work finding him a wife.

Choosing a mate in the Western district of Victoria, Australia, was easy enough. If a man found a woman who caught his fancy, he made no effort to court or impress her. Instead, he went to her father and asked his consent to the union. Her only choice was to run away if she did not want the man as her husband. If she did escape, she could be killed for the insult it caused him. A consolation was that the girl's family could, in all good conscience, avenge her death.

Ashanti girls were usually married off at birth. Often, they were promised as wives even before they were born. If for some reason the girl had no marriage possibilities while still quite young, she was displayed in a kind of parade. This advertisement usually yielded several offers of marriage.

Natives of the Trobriand Islands were married off by their parents while still babies. From childhood to adolescence, the couple were referred to as man and wife. They themselves spoke to and of each other as a married couple. Once of marrying age, at puberty, they were formally married.

The American Haidi Indians usually paired their offspring at a tender age. If the formal marriage was for some reason postponed, the Haidan boy took another girl. She lived with him as his wife until his original mate was ready.

The New Guinea Arapesh were paired with their partners very early in life. If a girl was not attached by the time she was 9, or at the oldest 10, she was an "old maid."

In some parts of India, it was an absolute necessity to have a daughter married off by the age of 12. Should the parents have not found a husband by the time she was a Rajasvala ("one who has experienced menstruation"), the whole family suffered. It was believed that the mother, father and oldest brother would to to hell if they had not married off their Rajasvala. As well, all their relatives would, every month, be forced to drink her menstrual blood.

In some cases, neither the marriageable girl nor her parents had a choice as to who her husband may be:

It was common among some tribes of India for a poor man, who could afford no dowry for his daughter, to take his daughter to the market. Banging his drum, he caught the attention of the people in the market. His daughter raised her dress in the back, then in the front, to expose herself and show off her charms to prospective husbands.

Among the Carib natives, a man chose his future wife by approaching a pregnant woman and painting her belly with a red cross. Should the woman deliver a daughter, it was understood that she was spoken for.

In some parts of northern Nigeria, a young girl was married off to the first man (other than relatives) who had seen her after she was born.

Among the Santal tribe of India, a man could claim a girl as his wife if he dabbed the girl on the forehead with red paint. This was not the usual method of acquiring a wife, and if a young man succeeded in doing so, the girl's parents were infuriated. But the man was still entitled to the girl, and the marriage had to be respected.

In many parts of the world, it has been the tradition that a father choose a husband for his daughter. However, some cultures respected her right to cancel a marriage to a partner she did not want:

It was rare that a Hottentot daughter disagreed with her father's choice of a mate. However, if she steadfastly refused, she was allowed to reject him, but only if she could keep her virginity by defending herself against the young man on her wedding night—with teeth, nails and fists.

It has been necessary, at times, to actually hire matchmakers:

Beginning in the Middle Ages, the Jewish people in Europe employed professional matchmakers. For the most part, these matchmakers were rabbis. They were called Shadkans, or Shadchans.
   These matchmakers were important to the survival of the race, especially in medieval times, when the systematic persecution and slaughter of the Jews made it difficult and dangerous for single men and women to make contact with each other.

In more advanced cultures, a woman being pursued by two lovers was allowed her choice. In more primitive societies, it has been a contest of two wills:

The two young Dongola men who wanted the same girl underwent a test of wills. The girl in question sat between the two lovers, holding two long knives in her hands at her sides. Slowly she pressed the knives into the thighs of the two young men. The last to move away won the hand of the girl.

Among the Slave Indians, two young men solved a romantic dispute over a girl by a test of strength. Each grabbed hold of the other's hair. The first to lose his grip lost the hand of the girl.

Among the Polynesians, if two young men were attracted to the same girl, the question was easily resolved. Each male took one of her arms and pulled until the other could no longer hold on to her. The man who could jerk the girl free from the other became her husband.

拭

Fathers have not been above choosing wives for their sons, for their own convenience:

Russian boys of the 18th and 19th centuries were promptly married at the age of 18. When possible, a father encouraged earlier marriage, so that he had another hand to share the work on the land. When this happened, the two youngsters were married, with the father entitled to perform the bedroom duties of his "underage" son. Once the boy turned 18, he was allowed sole sexual access to his wife.

拭

In rare instances, it has been the female's right to make the marriage match:

The Cantaberian Australian girl had the right and responsibility of picking a wife for her brother, giving the wife-to-be a dowry for marrying him.

The Wemba girl of South Africa was the initiator in the business of pairing off. If a boy turned down the girl's proposal, the girl's father was obligated to pay the boy a goat.

A Garos girl decided which man she wanted for a mate. It was a matter of manners, regardless of his wish, to turn the girl down, run and hide.
    The woman courting him would enlist his help to capture him. Most times he would escape a second time and be recaptured. If he ran away a third time, it was understood that he did not share the girl's feelings, and the proposal was forgotten.

Among a tribe called the Vizerees, inhabiting a mountainous area in India, a woman could propose to a man. She asked the tribe's drummer to attach her handkerchief to her lover's cap. The drummer did this in front of the whole village, and providing he could pay her dowry, the young man was obligated to marry the girl.

In India, a Kolarian girl who wanted a certain man for a husband went to his house and sat down inside. Her meaning was well understood, and he was obligated to marry her.

The Filipino Igorot girls and boys at puberty stayed in separate huts in the village. The girls were the pursuers in romance. A girl stole an item from a boy she liked during the day. This was an invitation to go to the girl's hut at night to reclaim his property, and, in the bargain, spend the night with the interested girl.

Superstition has influenced many a girl hoping to find her true love:

In ancient China, "the seventh day of the Seventh Moon" was of great significance to single girls. This was the ideal day to make wishes on future romance.

On the night of the seventh day of the Seventh Moon, girls would crawl under a square table and attempt to thread a needle in complete darkness—this threading being symbolically sexual. If she accomplished this, it was believed she would find a husband.

In North China, the ritual was a little different. On the evening of that day, the girls went into the darkness to pick cucumbers. A girl plucked the first cucumber she came upon, and rushed home to the privacy of her room to assess her future. The girl who picked a large and well-shaped cucumber was assured of finding her husband some time in the year. The girl who had the misfortune to pick an inadequate, misshapen cucumber was advised to wait the year out and postpone romance.

A Yugoslavian peasant girl, to make all men fall in love with her, carried a bat under her armpit.

Necessity has been responsible for taking old customs and reviving them. Advanced cultures have not been above borrowing from their ancestors:

Colonial Americans in the early 1600s celebrated the Maid's Fair. Male settlers in early America, in need of wives, paid the boat fare of their prospective wives to an enterprising businessman who ferried the strange women over. These women were not obligated to marry anyone that they did not wish to; however, inside the day of arrival, all were usually married off. There were many Maid's Fairs to come following the initial settlement, the custom lasting over 200 years.

The introduction of marriageable people has commonly occurred through public functions whose main aim was the pairing off of men and women:

The natives in Heilgherry practiced mass-mating. A fence through which nothing could be seen was built around a hut. Single women stood inside the hut, the males standing outside the fence, holding long sticks. The females left the hut one by one and grabbed one end of a stick. The two young people holding the same stick were married.

The Chinese of the Chou dynasty held festivals every spring, when many families migrated from their winter homes to the fields. These spring festivals celebrated the fertility of the land, and the hopeful fertility of the young men and women who paired off during the festival. The romance was enhanced by singing and dancing of an erotic nature. The relationship was consummated, and the couples were considered to have had a successful "encounter." The couple were encouraged to see each other through the summer and fall, although intercourse was not an assurance of a permanent match.

Some cultures had formal holidays that provided an opportunity to meet the opposite sex:

In England, and later in the United States, May Day was a day to find a mate. The cutting of the maypole provided a diversion to allow couples to go into the woods together. In 1583 Stubbs described this holiday, from which he claimed most of the girls came back sexually experienced:

> Against Maie, Whitsondaie, or other time, every parishe, town, and village assemble. They ran gadding to the woods and groves, hills and mountaines, where they spend all the night in pleasant pastymes, and in the morning they return, bringing home birch bowes and braunches. Their cheafest jewel they bring back home from thence is their maiepole, all covered with Flowers and Hearbes, with 200 or 300 Men and Women following it. And thus being reared up with handkerchiefs and flaggs streaming on the toppe. Then fall they to banquet and feast, to leape and daunce about, as Heathen people.

Koko-nor Tibetans were known to hold a hat-choosing festival called Tiao Mao Hui. The festival lasted three days. During that time the man went to the temple ground, looking for girls. When he found a suitable girl, the man removed her hat and took it home with him. That night the woman went to the male's hut, staying the night with the man to reclaim her hat and begin the relationship.

In ancient Ireland among the peasantry, it was the neighbors who decided when a young maid should be married. They also decided who the best match for her would be. After this was decided, they approached the girl and told her that she would be "horsed" the following Sunday.

On this particular Sunday, the girl provided refreshments, and all the eligible males drank the cider and whiskey and "horsed" the girl. That is, they carried the girl on their backs. This done, the young men proved their fitness and strength by engaging in a hurling match. Although she had her favorite chosen for her, if another young man won the hurling match, he could claim the girl as his bride-to-be.

In Ecuador, the Cayapan tribes frequently held fiestas. At some of these celebrations, the tribal leaders arranged marriages. Often the alcoholic gaiety broke down into pathetic, melancholy scenes. The men pressed into marriage lamented their circumstances as being unfit for marriage. They also argued that they were too young, too old, too busy or too poor to be married. This quickly took the joy out of the festivities.

The mating dance was and is a common prelude to the sexual connection. It inflamed passions and suggested and promised, through dance, the ecstasies of the sexual encounter:

The Minnetarees of North America practiced a mating dance. The females danced for about two hours before they accomplished their point. This dance consisted of waddling like ducks and removing one piece of clothing at a time. Once naked, they led their male counterparts to a private spot in the bush, and the mating dance's end was accomplished.

The Korani practiced a mating dance to encourage members of the opposite sex to courtship. A male danced in front of a number of females. Using his body language in a very suggestive manner, to all, then to each woman individually, he entertained them. Choosing his mate, he danced close around her. Then he jumped into her lap, whereupon they rolled on the ground with each other, the result usually being intercourse.

According to certain literature, women could get an indication of a man's virility without unclothing him:

Nicholas Venette, in his 18th-century manual of love, *The Mysteries of Conjugal Love Reveal'd*, stated that "Men with big Noses also have stout Members, and also that they are more robust and courageous than others."

Choosing a mate has inevitably come down to challenging and testing a mate's loyalty:

In southern India, the Gadaba girl was paired off with a young man. They then went off into the bush alone and built a fire. To test his courage, the girl took a burning stick and pressed it into her fiance's flesh. If he screamed, the pairing was canceled; if he did not, they had intercourse there and then, and the match was set.

Aitutaki women of the Cook Islands tested their lover's loyalty before they agreed to intercourse. The girl who wanted to assure herself of her lover's commitment did not wash her most private parts for several days. Then she demanded that her lover perform cunnilingus upon her. Having passed that trial, he was allowed to have intercourse with her.

The matter of sex in the pairing-off process has been a casual after-thought in many primitive cultures:

There was a high degree of sexual freedom among British New Guinea's Kiwi Papuans. While parents were unconcerned about their child's sexual activities, they nevertheless policed the children. Sexual experimenting and freedom was allowed, but a girl's parents wanted her to see only the proper boy: A boy who did not have a sister to trade for their daughter was not a welcomed boyfriend.

The Upper Tonkin Lolo tribe practiced casual mating. A couple spent a single night at a male's house, with the girl returning to her home afterward. She continued her erotic affairs with other young men, not obligated to any male she slept with.

If she happened to become pregnant and returned to a lover's house, they were considered married. Often, he was not the true father; this was understood, but usually did not affect his decision to marry her.

Yobai, or "night creeping," was practiced by the Japanese for centuries. After the rice-planting ceremonies, all the unmarried men got together for a party. After the party, the young men wandered about the village, looking for the houses of eligible young girls. These girls, with their parents' knowledge, kept their doors open to encourage the young men.

The group of boys played "scissors/paper/stone," or janken-pon. The boy who won janken-pon made his way into her room and they had sex. Then the group of boys moved quietly to the next house.

Often the young man urinated on the door to quiet the sliding of the door, and this was concrete evidence that the girl had already been visited. However, young women often had sex with more than one young man in the evening.

In Dalmatia, a young girl entertained two or three boys at night in the kitchen of her house. The next morning, after each had intercourse with her, they left. These kinds of parties happened until she became pregnant. She chose the boy she wanted as a father, and he was obligated to marry her. However, some girls did not always follow this line; often, a girl had two or three children in this way before she settled on marrying.

Among the Mexican upper classes, a boy wishing to get married practiced a random mating. The young man wanted to be sure his wife was fertile, so he paid a go-between to get a number of girls from good families. These girls were paid a small fee, then undressed and lined up in a row, crouching on their hands and knees. The young man had dog-style intercourse with each. However, he married only the girl who produced a son. The young man often had to go through this ceremony a dozen times to find a wife.

The sexual qualification for a mate was considered most important in some cases:

Among some Arab tribes, the woman did not accept a proposal of marriage until she closely examined the male's sexual parts.

Certain ancient Persian tribes had a custom whereby a man was not allowed to marry unless he had proved to his wife that he could sexually satisfy her. This required the husband-to-be to audition for his desired woman.

The Chibchas of the Andes in Central America scorned the idea of a girl retaining her virginity until marriage. They viewed a virgin as someone who must be either ugly or badly behaved, because it meant that apparently nobody had any interest in taking her virginity while courting her.

Many Australian aborigines secured possible mates only from other villages. A man waited for a dark, windy night and prowled around a foreign village, seeking a leubra, or female, who appeared eligible, sleeping by the fire. When he spotted her, he carefully twisted his spear into her long, thick hair, tangling the hair in the spear head. He then jerked the spear, waking her. He descended on her, knocked her senseless with his club and dragged her off. Once the kidnapped girl regained her senses, she was taken to the village of his people. There, he sexually forced himself on her, with the members of the clan looking on. In this way she was made his wife.

This rape ritual was a common occurence, and children of the villages, accustomed to this sort of mating practice, played "abduction rape" as a game. It was common that a very attractive Australian native girl could suffer through many abductions and rapes by bachelors from other villages.

An especially brave and skilled warrior who had kidnapped a girl would occasionally volunteer to undergo the "trial of spears." Ten of the best warriors from the tribe, having lost the woman, got three spears each. The lone warrior representing the kidnapping village held only a shield, and dodged and defended himself against the spears thrown. Having done this successfully, he was considered to have earned the right to his woman, and the two tribes held a great feast together.

Fiji Islanders and some New Guinea Papuans found wives by abducting and raping women from neighboring villages. It was only after the woman was in the foreign village and had been violated that arrangements were made to remedy the situation.

In the presence of holy men, the tribe she was abducted from was offered compensation for their loss by the abductor's tribe. The woman could return to her tribe, or stay in the new one, as she chose.

Because marriage has often been of more benefit to the community than to the individual, it is not surprising to find some people who have been relieved of the responsibility of courtship:

The southern Ecuadoran Cayapa man who remained single too long could count on having a wife picked for him. If the man had enjoyed being a bachelor or widower longer than the man's family thought proper, they contacted an eligible girl's family.

If it was agreed to by the woman's family, she left her people and went to the matchmakers to meet the male. The courtship was very short; he decided then and there whether he wanted her as a wife or not.

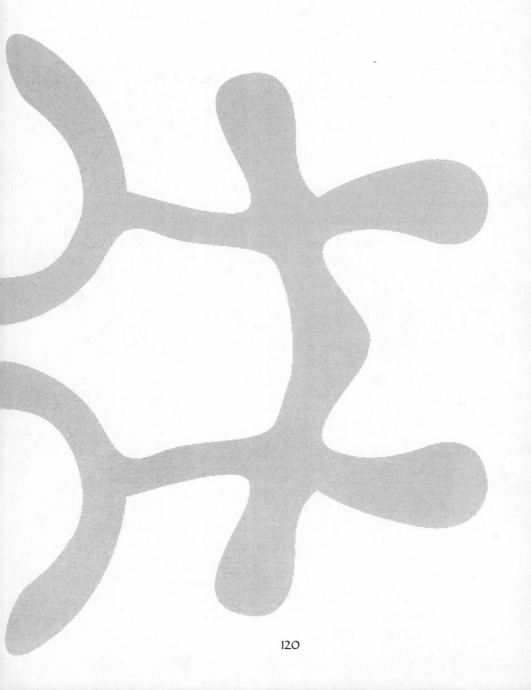

COURTSHIP

There have existed very noble, very idealized forms of love:

The chivalrous knight of the Middle Ages in Europe pledged his love to a lady while holding her hand. The knight then received a kiss for his devotion. He was given a single kiss each year he stayed loyal to his lady. This was the extent of the relationship. Any further gratitude shown was due only to the graciousness of the lady. Should a knight stay loyal but be deprived of her kiss, he could "sue" for it.

In the Heian age in Japan, the most valuable quality an eligible girl could have was her writing skill. Because the girl was not very socially visible, the young man interested in her usually had to write a letter declaring his interest. His declaration had to be well penned to stir her interest. For his part, her reply had to be poetic and subtle, and she had to show good penmanship. If she couldn't do this to his satisfaction, he didn't pursue her any further.

With these notes being passed back and forth by go-betweens, they rarely got a chance to see each other in the flesh. If they became interested in each other, the woman was as likely as the man to ask for a meeting. Visiting her late at night, the meeting, unlike the letters passed between them, was quick and to the point. The man merely came to the woman's bed and they had sex.

Given the literary nature of the courtship and meeting, it was not unusual for one of the partners to wake up the next morning with a bedmate who was not the person they had corresponded with.

The North American Crow Indian man often sought out a sexual partner at night. The young man crept around tents, searching for women's beds. Then he stuck his hands under the tent and tried to stimulate the girl's vagina. Once she was stimulated, he persuaded her to allow him to have sex with her.

While primitive people have often been thought to have sex without commitment, that has not always been the case:

The native women of New Zealand were not above having sex with mates they barely knew. However, there were certain manners involved, which made the sexual connection nearly as formalized as their marriages. The woman being courted insisted on receiving some tasty morsel as a sign of love for her in exchange for her sexual favors. As well, the connection had to be approved by all her girlfriends.

There have been varying standards by which cultures measured commitment:

In the Trobriand Islands, an unmarried girl who shared a meal with a boy was considered to have been more intimate with him than if they had indulged in sex.

The first men to show a sense of romance in courting were the troubadours of the mid-1600s. They introduced the concept of romance, the idea of winning a woman's heart through chivalry and good manners, quite unintentionally. The first French Troubadours began wandering about the countryside singing love songs to flatter women in exchange for food and lodging. All too often, the lady of the castle took the love songs very personally, resulting in unwanted affections, and, worse, hostility from the man of the castle.

Tenderness and courtesy have not always been the methods by which people have shown their love:

Somogyr women, though having received kisses, caresses and sexual favors from their men, did not believe that they were truly loved until they had received a good beating from their man.

While the age of chivalry was a turning point in the romance of love— as opposed to the economics—it was not completely free of the matters of money:

In the time of the troubadours, when courtly love as an ideal was the rage, it was reserved only for married women. Single women were not courted by the troubadours, who were too poor not to be "sponsored" by a married lady.

Declarations of love have not always been considered romantic:

In pagan Europe, love poems and love songs were regarded with the utmost horror. They were considered to be magic spells, and among the Nordic peoples, were punished as any other form of witchcraft was—with the death sentence.

In one way or another, a young man has always been required to prove his worth to his prospective in-laws:

An Eskimo man around Smith Sound in the Arctic was not allowed to marry unless he had killed a seal while courting.

The young Koyukuhtana man who had not yet killed a deer was thought to be physically incapable of producing children.

In medieval England, the young man who wanted to marry a girl went to her parents' house. He brought with him some wine.
   Should the parents have accepted the offer of a drink from it, he took their acceptance as their blessing regarding the marriage. Next, he squeezed an invitation to supper from them. If the girl served walnuts for dessert, the young man left; it was clear she did not want him.

The Yukaghir youth proved his worth to his prospective father-in-law by a test of strength. The girl's father went into the forest and cut down the tallest, largest tree. The young man was obligated to drag the tree back to his father-in-law's house and heave it onto the home. If he managed to dump the tree on the shelter and destroy it, the old man was satisfied. He was without a home but had found a strong son-in-law.

In some cases, societies have tested the economic benefit of certain pairings:

The Naga Hill tribe of Ao required that the courting couple set out on a 20-day business trip. If the trip was a material success, the couple married. If, however, it was a financial failure, no matter how well the couple got along, the marriage plans were abandoned, and they had to find other mates.

Often, the young man spent most of the courtship trying to get a father's blessing:

A young Laplander could visit his girlfriend as often as he wanted. However, there was one catch: Every time he visited the girl, he had to give her father a bottle of brandy as a token of his respect. Fathers, for this reason, did their best to postpone their daughters' wedding for as long as possible, and in any way they could.

The young Chukcha man interested in a girl was obligated to serve her and her family. No matter how wealthy he was, he was treated as a slave, ill-fed and abused by her family. No matter how high his reputation, he was obligated to perform the lowest chores until they regarded him as a worthy husband. Even if he had fathered her children, he was not assured her hand.

In South America, many of the native tribes had competitions among the bachelors wanting a girl's hand. The gentlemen interested in the girl were pitted against each other, usually for two or three years. In that time, they all worked for the girl's father, doing every kind of chore they were asked to perform. The most qualified and hardworking of the group was finally allowed to marry the girl.

The common courtship pattern in the world (if it can be said to exist) is that a male shows his affection and loyalty before he exhibits his sexual interest in a female. Of course, there are variations of this behavior to be found:

The Mangaian girl of the southern Cook Islands judged the strength of a boy's affection for her in one way. He had to, before anything else, approach her sexually and demonstrate his great and overwhelming desire for her body.

The sexual aspect of courtship has generally been large. In some cultures, the lack of sexual activity among courting couples was a source of amusement:

In 16th-century Brazil, the adolescent boy who did not show the scars from a case of syphilis was teased and abused by his lack of sexual experience with females.

The behavior of courting men and women has been almost always tender. Rare exceptions to this approach have existed:

The Basongye woman of the Congo who was interested in a male had an unusual way of showing it. It was the practice of a woman who was sexually attracted to a man to go to his house and strike up a conversation. This conversation, on the woman's side, consisted of a series of insults and putdowns toward the man. From her nasty words, the Basongye man could tell that she was in love with him.

When a Trobriand girl and boy desired each other, before they slept together, they indulged in Kimali. Kimali was the sign of affection a girl showed her man. Confident in his love for her, she was allowed to inflict any and all kinds of pain on her man.

To accomplish this, she beat, thrashed and cut him. He took this abuse cheerfully, knowing it was her love for him, and her desire to have sex with him, which made her do this.

Kimali Kaysa was the group form of Kimali. Dressed in festival costume, the single boys walked around a clearing, singing. Standing around the group of boys, the girls of the tribe teased and joked at the boys. Then they scratched, kicked and bit the young men. They attacked them with mussel shells, bamboo knives and even small, sharp axes. The boys welcomed the blows, knowing that later on they could claim a sexual reward from the girls who had abused them.

A very modern instance of this form of primitive custom has occurred:

In Spain in the 17th century, there emerged the practice of "sadistic courting." This mania was inspired by monks who scourged their flesh to punish themselves for lustful thoughts and keep themselves from feeling the stirrings of their bodies. It was now fashionable for courtiers to beat their flesh. The experts in this art, the clergy, gave lessons in how to do this properly. They even instructed on the mannered way of holding the rod and scourge.

During holy week, these lovesick flagellants took torchbearers and caroused the streets, then stopped below the balconies of the ladies they favored. They beat their flesh with the scourges, encouraged by the ladies. Sometimes they stopped to have their ladies favor them by tying ribbons around the instruments of punishment. This carnival of painful courtship was frequently followed by a feast.

Courtship could be subtle and slow, or obvious and quick to the point:

The man of the Crow Indian tribe made his desires to a woman clear by rubbing and playing with a woman's labia and clitoris.

The youth of the Wanigela River region of New Guinea displayed his interest in his chosen girl in a very indirect way. It was ill-mannered to talk to her or look at her. Instead, when he was in her presence, still ignoring her, he showed her his athletic skill, jumping, running and exercising to impress her. He even chased imaginary enemies away, throwing invisible spears at them.

On the island of Alor in the East Indies, the male indicated his interest in a woman by pulling her breasts. This made the woman so passionate that it was believed she could not refuse intercourse.

The Kurtatchi woman of the Solomon Islands made her desire to get to know a man very clear. Upon seeing him, she laid down in front of him with her legs open.

The use of magic to win a cold heart has been used even into relatively recent times:

The Tyroleans believed that if a man held a handkerchief under his armpit while he danced with his girl, then presented it to her, the handkerchief would make him irresistible to her.

In peasant Prussia, the male lover desiring to be paired with a particular woman searched the marshes for two frogs that were mating. While they were still stuck together, he inserted a needle through the pair and removed it. He then went to the woman he desired and pinned a piece of clothing to a part of hers using the needle. This made her fall in love with him forever.

The ancient Greek who wanted a woman to fall in love with him, used magic to help his cause. The magic formula: He tied a hyena's udder around his left arm.

In ancient Ireland, girls secured the love of the man of their choice in this way: The lovesick girl went to the graveyard at night and dug up a corpse which had laid there for nine days. She tore off a strip of skin from the corpse's head to the foot. She took this skin and wrapped it around the arm or leg of the man of her choice as he slept. She then removed it before he awoke and kept it in her possession. In this way the girl kept the love of her man, for as long as she kept the skin of the corpse.

Love potions were popular with the 19th-century French. One of the simplest of these potions was designed to win over a man. A woman simply gave the man of her choice a glass of wine mixed with a few drops of her menstrual blood.

The northeast African Siwan man ensured the love of a desired woman by using a love potion. He gave the woman some food mixed with his semen.

In central Sumatra, it was believed that a person could win another's love if they smeared elephant semen over the object of their desire. The semen, however, had to be taken from the elephant just before it was ready to have intercourse.

Some cultures were very tolerant of a courting couple's privacy:

Celtic and Germanic people in the pre-Christian ages had a custom called Maraichinage. On a certain evening once a week, commonly a Saturday, single girls kept their bedroom doors and windows open to the visits of bachelors. The admirers spent the night with their girls.

The couples were either fully or partially dressed. They talked, cooed, and slept in each other's arms. Intercourse was strictly forbidden. To ensure restricted dallying, bells were attached to the bed's legs. Often, the girls were bound above and below their knees with rope.

Holland in the 15th century was the location of the Questeen. On the island of Texel, houses had an opening under the window where lovers entered so that they could sit on the bed and spend the night making love to their girlfriends. The houses of Holland were built with this special entryway. A girl was seen as very coarse if she did not have this aid to courting.

A Persian couple practiced Bosah-bauzee, or "kissing and toying." The new lovers never removed their clothes but were allowed to touch and fondle without restraint. Attaining pleasure by fully clothed manipulation enhanced the desire and thus the pleasure of the two.

The female moved her body against the boy, stroking herself with his form, until she climaxed. The boy, as a proposal, kissed her between the eyes. Thereafter, she kept her distance. She was not seen by him until the wedding. If the girl died before she was wedded to her intended, her body was taken to the boy's house. A priest witnessed as the boy penetrated her for the first and last time, and she was then cremated.

In several cultures, the women had the initiative in choosing a partner:

Maori women showed their sexual interest in a man by scratching or pinching the palm of his hand. This was an unmistakable sexual invitation.

It was the female of the Radeh people of southern Indo-China who pursued the male. She sent a male friend to propose the match to the man of her choice. If the man was agreeable, she moved into his parents' house for a year. While there, she seduced the man, hoping to become pregnant. If she did, she was obligated to pay a dowry to his parents in cloth or cattle, before she could take him away.

Ancient Egyptian women were the sexual aggressors in their time. The men of that period took great pleasure in playing at shyness and were very coy. They encouraged and forced the ardent women to chase them. They also delighted in being taken advantage of by having the women get them drunk on wine.

The Hopi girl of northwest Arizona proposed to the boy. The wedding announcement was provided by her combing his hair in public.

In the Kamchadale tribe, the female was dominant. Women pursued the males of their choice, to the point of physically fighting over them. Once married, the men were no less passive. Demand or reason could not persuade their wives to get or do anything the women did not want to do. The men pleaded, begged and traded their affections to get what they desired from their wives.

The girl of the Melanesian Banks Islanders chose a man who interested her and pursued him. But it was not he whom she asked when she wanted to take the relationship further. Instead, she went to one of his aunts and asked her permission to have sex with him.

The Assam's Khasi tribe girls were the pursuers in the courtship process. It was understood that the males must resist their advances at every turn. This coyness reached a climax when the man she was chasing actually ran away. The girl, with help, trapped her man and returned him to the village and her house. His parents cried, as was the custom, and mourned for their newly wedded son.

The South American Goajiro girl who was interested in a boy tried to trip him during the ceremonial dance. If she succeeded and he fell to the ground, it was her right to have sex with him.

Envious older folk could turn innocent courting into humiliation:

It was common in medieval France for a couple innocently courting in public to be accused of adultery. Lovesick couples merely embracing or kissing were accused of having sexual relations.

When looking for a little entertainment and fun, bored villagers often picked on a courting couple for their amusement in this way. The locals of the village often wrongly accused a pair of adultery for the simple fun of seeing them punished for their "crime." The punishment usually took the form of parading the couple through the town's streets naked, while teasing and abusing them.

The simpler cultures of the world, free from complicated social structures and obligations, dealt with the question of sex in courtship plainly:

Among some tribes of North American Indians, a young man wanting to spend the night with a girl entered her hut with a stick. He lit the stick from her campfire, and if she blew it out, he stayed the night. If she put the bedcovers over her head, he left, having been rejected.

To proposition a girl he was interested in having sex with, the Pacific Tikopia man flipped up her skirt.

The South American Siriono couple spent their time courting very efficiently. They picked lice out of each other's hair, and picked wood ticks from their partners' bodies, eating them. They picked worms and thorns from each other's skin, decorated each other with feathers and paint, then had sex.

A night of romance, as described by a Trobriand male: "We walk, we arrive at a large tree, we sit down, we search each other's heads and eat the lice, we tell the woman we want to have sex. After it is over, we return to the village."

The Jaluit man of the Marshall Islands indicated his desire for intercourse with a girl by saying "penis" and "vagina" and suggestively rolling his eyes.

A Dahomean woman of the west coast of Africa showed her interest in a man by dropping her skirt and exposing herself.

Among the Congolese, sex was a natural part of courtship, and all were expected to participate. Their word for "virgin" had the same meaning as "idiot" or "fool."

In some cultures, courtship did not feature the usual male-female roles:

When their use as warriors was taken away, the Tchambuli men became dependent on their women, who supported the tribe by weaving and fishing. The men became "feminine"—dependent, artistic, and more emotional than their mates. Their role was now to be amusing. The men spent their time in games and theatrical offerings for the women. On holidays, these citizens of the Amazon dressed like their women, as a signal to courtship.

Virginity has not been a common requirement of many eligible young people:

Often, the Samoan girl did not or could not get out of the house at night to meet her lover. Sometimes she would announce this. If her lover wanted her company, he had to visit her in her parents' hut while they were asleep. This boy was known as Moetotolo, "the sleep crawler." He did this by removing the Lavalava from his body and greasing himself with coconut oil. The oil was to prevent anybody from getting a good grip on him, should he have to escape. He then silently entered the girl's hut.

Taking advantage of this plan, the boy might crawl into a girl's hut, even though she did not expect him. He took the chance that she might or might not accept his sexual favors and reveal him to her family. If the girl decided not to accept the boy's sexual advances, she sounded the alarm. When this happened, it was great sport, and the females of the hut, feeling the most threatened, gave the best chase to this young "thief."

The Yungar boy of southeastern Australia carried a "love rod"—a carved walking stick. Each stick was uniquely carved. At night, a boy would go to a girl's house and thrust the stick through the hut's wall, nudging her. Once she identified the young man by his trademark stick, she could allow or deny him access to the hut to have sex.

In ancient China, the girl who kept her virginity to age 17 was considered something of a freak. To cure this embarrassment, a boy was hired. The girl took off her clothes, grabbed hold of a pillar in the house and bent over. The boy took her virginity with neither one ever seeing the other's face.

In parts of Germany, premarital sex was very common, and no shame was attached to indulging before marriage. It was a common custom for the female, once faced with the chance to have sex with her lover, to initiate a wrestling match with her lover. If her man overpowered her, she gladly had sex with him. But if she proved stronger than him and he could not take her by force, she laughed him away, and their relationship was over.

There was a good deal of sexual entertaining by the Akambans of East Africa. Frequent sex with many different partners was common. In fact, it did not upset the Akamba boy to visit his lover, only to find that he had been replaced sexually by his lover's girlfriend.

Premarital sexual restrictions have not necessarily been a sign of a sexually "moral" society:

In East Africa, among the Rundi, the Hutu and Tutsi, sexual freedom before marriage was forbidden. There were serious punishments for a girl's premarital sexual adventures. Once they were married, however, the girls were allowed to have sex with any and all men they had flirted with when they were single. Their husbands seemed to care little about this change.

There was no objection to premarital sex as far as the East African Nandi were concerned. The only stumbling block to premarital sex was pregnancy. The child of an unmarried couple was automatically killed. The mother was forbidden to look at any of the tribe's granaries, because it was believed that the woman who had suffered this misfortune would spoil the grain inside it with just one look.

Native girls of the Dutch East Indies were free to sleep with the men of their choice as soon as they reached the age of maturity. Because of the girl's absolute freedom, the men did everything they could to secure a promise of marriage from their desired girl. They did not want their fellow tribesmen to have sexual knowledge of their girlfriends.

The Bukumatula, or young people's lodge, was common in New Guinea. Once the search was successful, the lucky boys and girls explored the matter in the Bukumatula. Young couples made temporary arrangements to live together in these Bukumatulas. Most of the "living" however, was spending the evening and night together having sex. During the day the young couple lived with their separate families.

This home away from home was perfect for exploring the erotic possibilites of the relationship. But the sexual attention was not restricted to familiar couples; everyone was fair game, whether she or he had a partner or not.

The couples could stay together for several nights. There was one firm rule, however: The couple could not eat together.

The marriage proposal has almost universally been the responsibility of the man. This has not always been the case:

In the Torres Straits and southern Papua, in New Guinea, girls were the only ones allowed to propose marriage. Part of the puberty rites among the young men of the area featured a very stern lecture warning boys against proposing marriage to girls.

Once proposed to, the young man was never eager to answer. He was taught that the girl must ask for his hand in marriage several times, so that he could determine whether or not she was really serious about him.

The height of courtship, the proposal, was often a simple, symbolic gesture:

The courting gentleman of ancient Ireland proposed to his intended by offering her a bracelet of his braided hair. To accept the bracelet was to accept the man in marriage.

The ancient Persian Medes couple announced their engagement by going to a public place and cutting each other's arms. They each contributed their blood to a cup, then drank the mixed blood.

The southeastern Australian Kamilaroil native men proposed marriage in a simple way. The man offered a woman food. If she accepted, they were engaged.

The Kurnai woman of southeastern Australia proposed to the man of her choice by asking, "Will you give me some food?"

The proposal in Caracas was a very simple affair. The male who desired a certain female told her of his wish to have her. He then went to her home. Should she have shown up while he waited there for her, he followed her into her hut. If she allowed him to wash himself in her basin and fed him, he could assume that she was willing to marry.

The proposal now accepted, they finalized their arrangement with their first sexual encounter. He was not allowed to divorce her for any reason. If she did not wish to stay with him anymore, for any reason, she had only to tell him to leave. Both were free to remarry afterward.

In Scotland a young man's proposal followed this routine: His young lady was sent to the local tavern. The young woman knew what to expect when this was done, and dressed in her finest clothes. He bought her a glass of ale and asked if she would have him. She answered.

If she said yes, he replied that he had heard from others that she would refuse him. She replied by saying that they were liars. He asked again, and she said that she had agreed twice already. Then the two licked the thumbs of their right hands and pressed them together, declaring their loyalty to each other. By doing this they were formally engaged.

A young man in 19th-century Dinan, France, proposed by giving his sweetheart a good slap on the knee during a local dance and asking, "Have you got another like this, *coquine*?" To encourage him, her reply was "Feel and see."

Then, a few days later, the young man would ask her, "Well, do you want to be the mother of my brats?" That settled, they treated each other quite formally during the engagement. They attended the county fairs together, holding each other by their little fingers.

In Bretagne, France, and neighboring areas in the late 1800s and very likey long before, the customary way of proposing marriage was for the potential bride and groom to spit into each other's mouths.

In Serbia and Bulgaria, among the peasants, a man proposed to a woman by simply grabbing her by the ankle and tripping her to the ground.

There have been forms of courtship that greatly resembled the married state, or entitled the couple to the advantages of marriage:

The Arapesh people of New Guinea paired off girls of about seven to young men approximately 13 years old. They lived together for several years not as true husband and wife, but more as brother and sister. When the girl came of age to have sex, they then truly became husband and wife.

In New England in the 18th century, a woman could enjoy the status of being married without the actual ceremony or full commitment. It was actually a premarriage commitment. In this condition, she was technically single but viewed as married to her lover. In fact, if she was caught having sex with a man other than her "steady," she was charged with adultery.

The custom of "tarrying," or waiting in expectation, occurred in the 18th century. The young man living in the American colonies notified his sweetheart's parents that he intended to marry her. With their consent, the man tarried for the night. Should the result of their union not have been as satisfying as they expected, they were both free to go their own ways.

In ancient Japan, after the first night spent together (the man had to sneak into his lover's room), there was an exchange of poems and letters. Then there was what was known as the Second Night. They again spent the night in the woman's room (he again having to sneak in), expressing their love. This time, however, there was more of a commitment to each other. On the Third Night, the understanding was that they were to be married, and he did not have to sneak into her room.

He presented himself to her parents and they shared rice cakes and sake, or rice wine. If she was not his first wife (who was entitled to a big wedding), the exchange of sake cups symbolized their union. The Third Night was considered their wedding night. The next morning the new son-in-law did not have to slip out, and the Fourth Morning was a relaxed, leisurely one.

The locality of Portland, England, had this custom as late as the 19th century: The girls of the region did not usually marry until pregnant. A Portland girl lived faithfully with her lover, and married only when she gave birth to a child. If she lived with him an unusually long time without becoming pregnant, the couple considered it something of a warning that the relationship would not work, and they parted company.

During the 18th century, the New England Puritans courted through a "courting stick." The couple sat in the parents' cabin, in full view of the family. The male and female sat on either side of the fireplace, with the courting stick running between them. The courting stick was between six and eight feet long and an inch or so in diameter. It was hollowed out. The couple spoke to each other through this long tube, whispering sweet nothings to each other.

Marriage

The ancient Persian who died a virgin was married before burial. The person marrying the corpse was paid for this service.

In Sweden, before and for quite some time after Christianity made its appearance, the bride on her way to her wedding was often kidnapped, taken as a ready bride by her kidnappers. With the increase of this practice, weddings became armed affairs. Then, to aid in security, the wedding was held at night. For this night ceremony, custom-made lances were created, with torch holders attached to them.

For a very long time, marriage was, in the main, widely a matter of buy, sell and trade:

When a young Malaili man of southern India wished to get married, his father set off to other villages to find a suitable wife. At each village he stopped at, he asked as to the availability of a bride. He agreed to take the girl chosen by a four-member council of the village he visited.

The Australian Dieri, as well as other neighboring tribes, negotiated marriages between the tribes. These negotiations could last several months. Gifts of weapons and tools were sent to the chief of the tribe, as well as to his important lieutenants, and the bride's father. The bride received nothing, except a husband. Neither of the youngsters was consulted on who they might prefer to marry.

In ancient China, family negotiations were entered into once a match was set. The engagement was set, and the number of presents agreed upon between the two families. Once a marriage contract was established, it could not be broken. If the bride's friends opposed the marriage, the person responsible for giving her away was beaten with a bamboo cane 50 times, but the marriage went ahead. If the bridegroom or his friend became unhappy about the match before the wedding, the dissatisfied person was also beaten with 50 strokes of the bamboo—and the marriage went on.

In Germany during the 16th century, the trade guilds monitored the character of the women who became involved with their membership. The woman who was to be married to a tradesman had to be formally introduced to the membership at a meeting, where her character was carefully questioned. If the marrying man did not bring her to this prenuptial meeting, he was thrown out of the association.

When a young man approached an Abandian mother about marrying her daughter, he was directed to her brother. Each girl had a brother "for whom she was born"; it was he who decided who she married. It was also he who received her dowry.

A Banyoro man of Central Africa who was too poor to pay cattle for his wife could take her on credit. The groom was allowed to pay on installments if he was not rich enough to cover the bride-price. To keep him honorable, it was practice that his children belonged to his father-in-law until his wife was paid for. The children could be returned to their father for one cow and, of course, the balance of the bride-price.

In Greece, from the time of Christ, a woman came with a dowry for her husband. If a girl did not have parents to provide a dowry for her, her closest male relative had to provide one, or marry the girl himself.

Parents in ancient Wales lent their daughters out to young men interested in marrying. The young man paid for this trial engagement. If he did not marry the girl, on returning her to her parents he also had to pay them an extra fee.

The Sumatran males of Indonesia practiced buying wives with another female as exchange. A man sold his sister, and if without a sister, a cousin. It often happened that the groom even borrowed a female from a friend, promising repayment at a later date.

Among many tribes of North American Indians, women taken as prisoners were married into the tribe. A warrior traded a woman he had captured to one of his friends who had also captured a female. If the man could not trade them off, he gave them away, because the warriors were never allowed to marry the girls they themselves had taken prisoner—it would have been incestuous.

Should a woman have lost her husband in battle, she was given a male prisoner. He automatically became a full member of the tribe, with all its rights and responsibilities.

A South African Wemba man paid a dowry for his wife. If the wife died or was unable to fulfill all her wifely duties, the man could choose one of her younger sisters to take her place.

In eastern Mongolia, the marriage bargain between families was not settled in the privacy of the home. The agreement was struck in the marketplace, with many of the relatives of both families haggling, for several days, as to the terms of the union.

In ancient Assyria, girls of marriageable age were considered the property of the state. Once a year girls were taken to the marketplace, and the choicest were sold to the highest bidder. Some of the money received from the sale of the attractive girls was put into a pot, and some money was offered to the buyers of the uglier girls.

Zulu wives were often very moneywise and enthusiastically helped their husbands to build a fortune. The woman worked very hard to secure a nice nest egg. This was because the first wife eagerly awaited her husband's purchase of a second wife. Far from being jealous, the first wife looked forward to having a junior to order around and perform the harder and less pleasant chores around the household, as well as the elevated status of being a senior wife. It was then that she passed on the more tiring chores to the younger wife.

The Chukchee woman who became too old for her husband's taste was either made a servant to his younger wives or forced to leave the household.

Among the northern Albanians, Montenegrins, and western Balkans, girls could escape an unhappy pairing by becoming "sworn virgins." These girls were obligated never to have intercourse with a man. The penalty was death. They lived out their lives dressing and drinking and smoking, acting as men, performing all the duties of a man and indulging in drinking and smoking, activities reserved only for men.

Marriage has been viewed as a way in which society could be maintained by legally ordered relationships. But in the interests of saving a society, priorities could change:

During the Peloponnesian War, the monogamous Greeks were faced with a crisis. Athens' population was devastated by military losses and plagues. The only solution was to promote the marriage of two women to every man.

In some instances, marriage was regarded as a necessary institution, but very imperfect romantically:

The Court of Love of the Middle Ages in Europe adjudicated lovers' disputes. Typical of the romantic thinking of the time was this statement by the "magistrate," the Countess of Champagne, concerning a case heard on May 3, 1174: "Love cannot exist between married people for the reason that lovers grant everything unconstrainedly, whereas married people are obliged to submit to one another."

The vast majority of cultures, past and present, throughout the world have promoted marriage. There are few cultures that did not promote it:

The ancient Greeks generally had little taste or use for marriage, and at one time it was more common to legally adopt a woman than to marry her.

Marriage came to be so unpopular in ancient Greece that the Athenian Solon was forced to pass laws promoting marriage. Important government posts were to be filled only by married men. It was hoped that if for no other reason than to further their careers, men would marry.

Men were sexually ignoring their wives in favor of other women, and this neglect of wives caused a booming market for dildos. In the sixth century B.C., to discourage adultery and reduce the number of men taking up with other men's wives, Solon was forced to make prostitution a state interest. He was instrumental in setting up a huge, low-priced, government-owned whorehouse in Athens.

The Greek Hesiod (8th century B.C.) said this of marriage: "He who evades, by refusing marriage, the miseries that women bring upon us, will have no support in the wretchedness of his old age. On the other hand, he whose fate it is to marry may perhaps find a good and sensible wife. But even then he will see evil outweigh good all his life." Further, Hesiod advised this method of setting up a household: "Get yourself first of all a house, a woman, and a working ox. Buy the woman, don't marry her. Then you can make her follow the plough, if necessary."

The children of a marriage could often be considered commercial property:

It was a common occurrence among the Romans to place children against their father's debts. They were often used in this way as security against a debt.

There have been instances in which a marriage hysteria has occurred:

When World War I broke out in France, couples who were living together and not legally bound flocked to have their unions formalized. With the uncertainty of life before them, thousands of couples rushed to get married. Magistrates' clerks received thousands of couples, and with so many requests in so short a time, often married 20 couples or more in a single mass ceremony.

In some parts of Paris, mass-marriages of as many as 300 couples were performed.

Premarriage requirements have been necessary in some areas of the world:

The Guayquiry bride-to-be of Orinoco had to fast for 40 days before her wedding.

The girls in several tribes in Africa, including the Nigerian Ibos, before married, were sent to "fattening houses." In these places they were gorged with food to make them more beautiful for the marriage. If they disappointed by not gaining the expected amount of weight, they were beaten.

On a French expedition to South America's Maroni River, Dr. Crevaux discovered this premarriage custom:

> About a hundred vicious ants are applied to the chest of such candidates and allowed to sting them. Enormous wasps are then made to attack their foreheads. Finally the young men are left in their hammocks for two weeks, almost without food, and writhing in pain. Beneath them a small fire of green wood is carefully left burning, so that a steady stream of acrid smoke will rise into the youth's nostrils. It is thus that they are prepared for the joys of marriage.

The obligation the bride had in entering a marriage may in some cases have been equally demanding:

Ancient Phoenicians, Lydians and Etruscans practiced the prostitution of engaged women. The women prostituted themselves to earn a dowry to give to their husbands, or to ward off evil spirits which might harm the union. In some cases, it was a "sacrifice" to the gods of love and fertility.

The oldest method of committing to marriage was by the male buying his bride:

The Ossete man who wanted to marry was obligated to present every member of his expected bride's village with a gift of money.

The heathen Anglo-Saxon wedding vows were worded in almost exactly the same terms as another legal function—the transfer of land.

Financial considerations have been a major factor in the pairing of men and women. However, other considerations could overrule this:

In ancient Rome, a marriage could not be made until an animal was sacrificed and its stomach and bowel contents examined; if no bad signs were found, the marriage was undertaken.

It has not been unusual for a groom to marry more than once, as a matter of custom:

Before a Kurmi man entered into matrimony, to confuse the gods of bad luck and not curse his wife, he was first required to "marry" a mango tree.

In southern India it was common that the Brahamian brothers marry in order of birth. Older brothers always married before younger ones. When the elder brother's prospects did not look good, the younger was allowed to marry a girl beforehand. However, to satisfy the requirement, the senior brother was first married off—to a tree.

Christian marriage has not always been a church ceremony. Though it was delegated to the church, it was, for a very long time, not performed in the place of worship:

Starting in the fourth century and continuing for over six centuries, marriages were performed in a ceremony outside the church doors.

The evolution of Christian marriage has been chaotic. The customs and ceremonies of the past do not resemble the modern affair. Sometimes marriage was a seasonal ceremony:

At one point in medieval England, only one half of the year was allowed for marriage; outside of this particular time, it was prohibited.

⚥

Eastern cultures have been well known for their inclination to marry at an early age. But the Western world has also followed this policy:

In medieval England, the age at which a couple could marry without their parents' consent was seven.

In 16th-century England, it was not uncommon for children to be married. In fact, in the mid-16th century, James Bullard, age 10, married a girl in Colne after she'd offered him two apples to marry her.

⚥

There have been different ways in which the bride and groom showed affection for each other:

In France of the Middle Ages, once the marrying couple exchanged vows, they exchanged small gifts. Then, as a sign of tenderness, they shook hands. Sometimes they might even kiss.

An alternate form of showing true commitment on the man's part was for him to hold her in his arms and declare, "So that you won't think I'm just taking advantage of you, I put my tongue in your mouth in the name of marriage."

⚥

In parts of England in the early 18th century, a newly married couple had a cake broken over their heads.

⚥

Among the Yukaghir, the bride was decorated in a very symbolic manner for her wedding ceremony. She was smeared with blood.

⚥

In the first century B.C., the ancient Briton woman showed up for her wedding dressed in her finest clothes. The groom attended his wedding absolutely nude.

⚥

Marriage ceremonies have, in a large part, been based on symbolic gestures:

Among the Scottish Gypsies, a highly symbolic ceremony took place. The priest took the marriage bowl and handed it to the bride. The bride squatted and urinated into the bowl. Then the priest gave the groom the bowl to urinate into. Then he mixed in some soil, and in some cases brandy. Both the bride and the groom were then asked to try to separate the mixture. They were told that, like this mixture in the marriage bowl, they were now inseparable.

The custom of having a best man at the wedding is very old, and found among primitive and modern cultures throughout the ages. While he serves in more recent times as a witness, originally the best man was picked as the friend most fit to help the groom capture the bride. Many cultures featured marriage by kidnapping, and in many more, the bride, groom and both families pretended that the girl was abducted. Often, the "grief" and "anger" shown seemed very realistic.

For instance, among the Indian Gonds, the young man took his intended on his back, from her village to his. His friends served as bodyguards, while the girl's friends pelted the wedding party with sticks, stones and abuse. Once the newlyweds reached his village, the bride's girlfriends were sent on their way, and the couple settled in.

The best man was usually called on to hold off, either in real style or in symbolic manner, the family members who came to the bride's rescue. The aspect of capturing the bride has, for the most part, disappeared, but the tradition of the best man continues.

A very old and widespread custom in England was that of the guests and relatives throwing their footwear at the bride and groom. The reason behind this ritual is obscure. Perhaps it was the symbolic clash of the relatives with the man or woman who was stealing their family member away, at a time when the groom abducted the girl to make her his bride.

The wearing of the wedding ring on the left hand is symbolic of the willingness of the mate to submit to his or her partner. The left hand has always taken the meaning of submission, while the right is the hand of supremacy and rule.

Brides and grooms in Elizabethan England wore their wedding rings on their thumbs.

In Portugal, the officiating "priest" tied the couple's hands together with a piece of his clothing.

About the time of the Middle Ages, in France, as a part of the marriage ritual, the bride let the wedding ring fall to the ground, then stooped in front of her husband to get it back.

In medieval France, the marriage ceremony was closed by the new bride kissing her husband's foot. Sometimes the ceremony of submission had a variation; he deliberately stepped on her foot.

In Russia, among the peasant population, part of the marriage ceremony involved the bride removing her husband's boots, and the groom giving her a sound beating.

☿♂

Marriage has been a sober, pious ceremony—most of the time:

The groom in the Babar Islands had to find his bride in a hut that was made pitch dark. The bride, if shy, could make this search a long one.

In Transylvania, the groom had to "pick" his bride from behind a curtain. In addition to his loved one, however, were several of her female relatives, including her grandmother.

Among the Indians of the Elk Nation, at the annual feast, "matrimonial mounds," high plots of dirt, were built up around which circular trails ran. She started at one end of the track, he at the other. She had to run around the mounds three times at top speed. If he caught up with her before the end of her circuit, he married her on the spot. If not, he was not allowed to take her as his wife.

In Germany, the peasant bride showed her partner that she expected an equal say in the household. She did this by constantly insisting that she have the upper hand when the priest joined their hands. The groom, for his part, resisted, and each jostled for the position of superiority in the handhold.

In northern England, it was customary for male guests to rush the bride at the altar when the wedding ceremony was over. The rush was to remove the garter from her leg. Usually this panic meant that the bride was knocked over and trampled on.

Gradually, brides made the garters easier to detach, and finally, to avoid any threat of injury, they tossed their garters away at the end of the ceremony.

☿♂

An important ceremony such as marriage has always attracted much superstition:

In the Philippines, the marriage ceremony was concluded by having the priest take the bride's and groom's heads and knock them together.

In the Chatham Islands, it was absolutely essential that every relative of the Moriori bride and groom witness the wedding.

If any relative, no matter how distant or disliked, did not see the ceremony or take part in the wedding feast, that particular person had the right to annul the marriage.

In Tibet, the citizens practiced group-marriage. The marriage was made holy by splashing the bride with yak grease.

The Hottentot bride and groom knelt in front of the holy man who married them. At the end of the ceremony, the "priest" urinated on the married couple.

In some areas of China, the holy man officiating the wedding, to secure the union, tied the couple's hair together.

Among a Moorish tribe near the Sahara Desert in Africa, a single man attending a wedding was favored by having a bowl of the bride's urine splashed in his face.

Weddings during the Renaissance in France were very often held at night. The French believed that the evil spells cast on the couple were least effective in the nighttime. The spell the newly married couple feared the most was the Tying of the Laces—which would prevent the newly-weds from consummating the marriage. A cure, however, was available. For nearly 300 years, to prevent the Tying of the Laces, French grooms took the precaution of urinating through their wedding rings.

It was considered good luck for a Bakitara princess to urinate during her wedding ceremony. However, if she also had a bowel movement, she was the object of shame. In some cases, the shame of the family obligated them to kill the bride.

Once a bride in Brittany left the church, she made a cut under her breast. The groom then consumed some of her blood.

In 16th-century France, a newly married couple was obligated to stand outdoors in the nude while performing a curious ritual. To ensure the fertility of the union, the groom kissed the big toe of his bride's left foot. Each partner gave the other the sign of the cross with their heels, then with their hands.

In the 18th and 19th centuries in England, and in the United States in New England, it was believed that if a woman was married in the nude, her new husband was not responsible for her debts. It was rea-soned that since she brought absolutely nothing to her new husband, her debts were not his to assume either.

Some marriage ceremonies have not been without peril:

The Transcaucasian people, the Migrelians, confirmed their vows of marriage by having the man bite his bride on her breast.

In some Arab tribes, the marriage ceremony included a circumcision rite. It was the bride's honor to remove her groom's foreskin. But the surgery did not stop there. Skin on the shaft of the penis, as well as some tissue, was also removed.

Once the skin was peeled off, the blood was sprinkled over the bride's clothes. The groom was expected to show no pain; otherwise, his wife would question his masculinity. Later that night, the bride expected him to perform passionately and vigorously, regardless of the pain involved in gaining erection and entry with a raw penis.

Some marriages have been short on ceremony but highly symbolic affairs:

In North Wales, peasants were married in a very simple manner. A birch broom was leaned across the doorway of a peasant home. The young groom jumped over the broom and through the doorway. His bride followed afterward. Should the broom have fallen over, or if one of the couple had touched the broom, the marriage was not considered "legal."

The marriage ceremony between the South American Yurakare husband and wife was a simple procedure. The bride's godmother threw the bride to the ground. Then the godfather threw the groom on top of the bride.

Polynesian Islanders involved themselves in the groom's approach to the bride. The groom walked from his hut to the bride's hut. He did not walk on the ground. Instead, his friends and relations lay face down on the ground, and he walked on their backs. After having arrived at his bride's hut, he sat on a chair. This was a human chair, formed by a cluster of three old women.

In some cultures, the bride or groom did not attend their own wedding:

In southern India, the Mysorian Lambadis did not allow any males to witness the marriage of a couple, with the exception of the Brahman priest. Even the groom was absent.

The bride of the Ja-Luo tribe of the Upper Nile was entertained by her new brother-in-law at his house, and then a feast with all the relatives was held. The groom was absent during all these festivities.

Among some Polynesian tribes, the couple to be married did not go through the marriage rites. Instead, their mothers exchanged blood and were the ones between the two families who were actually "married."

The Estonian groom went through the marriage ceremony without his bride by his side. Instead, his brother took her place, dressed as the bride.

While weddings have commonly celebrated the coming together of two people, not everyone needed to know who the wedding was for:

In ancient Greece, the Massalias held a wedding with a bride, but no groom. At the feast were bachelors who had been invited to the celebration. After the wedding feast was over, the bachelors presented themselves, in a line, to the bride. She presented a gold cup of wine to the man she desired for her husband.

Marriage by abduction has been practiced in nearly every part of the world, at some time:

The Cayapan Indian males of southern Ecuador practiced two forms of getting a woman. They either approached the girl and proposed, or they approached the girl by "night-crawling." This involved approaching a girl at night in her parents' hut. It was called supu tangahimu, "stealing a woman." The man who secured a girl this way was very much admired.

The tradition of a symbolic struggle by the family to keep their daughter from being taken as a bride, and of the groom's family to wrest her free, has been enacted frequently. Marriage ceremonies and courtships have long been either violent or symbolically violent:

The Calmuck girl was helped onto a horse by her family, and she fled her village. The lover, in due time, chased her on his horse. If he could not catch her, he could not marry her. However, if he caught her, they had their first marital intercourse on the spot and returned to the village as husband and wife.

In northern Bantu, the Banyankole groom went to his bride's parents' hut to perform a ceremony. Inside the hut, his bride waited for him to be led in. He took her hand and led her to a cluster of relatives—the bride's and the groom's respective relatives. The two groups faced each other, and the groom directed his bride to a spot between the two groups.

A family member from the bride's side brought out a rope and tied it to her left leg, with lengths of rope left on each side of her limb. The tug of war between the families was long and vigorous.

Marriage initiations are not uncommon around the world:

The ancient Germanic peoples held weddings that were also testing grounds for the groom's courage. The wedding was a perilous exercise. The laws of Frisia stated that should the groom be murdered during the marriage ceremony, the bride could collect part of his estate only if she followed the corpse back to his home.

In Maranhao, the groom of the Capiekran Indians underwent a test before the end of his marriage ceremony. After all other ceremonies were done, the groom had to show his courage. Sitting in a gourd was a nest of stinging-ants who had been collected and starved. The groom scooped the ants up, and as they devoured his hand, he was obligated not to lose his nerve. If he did this, his marriage was sealed.

Among the Hanran Arabs living around the Nile, the groom was severely tested at his wedding. The young groom, as a test of strength, was whipped by his in-laws. If he could bear this with dignity, he passed the test, and shrieks of admiration from all the females present were his reward.

The Arab groom of Djeezan was circumcised just before his marriage ceremony. If he screamed or moaned or even showed signs of pain on his face, the bride-to-be could refuse to marry him.

In the Marche district of medieval France, the bride-to-be had sex with every man she met on the way to the church.

In some instances, the girl was left to fend for herself: Marrying a girl on the east coast of Greenland was painful for her. The male merely grabbed her by the hair or other suitable handle. He dragged her over to his hut, and the formality was over. These occasions were often noisy and quite violent. The man paid little attention to her discomfort.

For her part, to preserve her reputation, she had to energetically resist, showing extreme modesty. This usually resulted in her suffering more pain, as it only made the losing battle longer. There was no outside interference through all this, although the custom usually drew an interested crowd.

The Kirghiz allowed the young lovers of a girl of the village to form a hunting party. They then set out to pursue the girl of their choice. She was pursued through the woods by the party but was armed with a large whip. If the man who approached her in the course of this chase was not a man of her choice, she used the whip on him.

The Bedouin girl of the Sinai was often not given a choice of whom she wished to marry. Her father arranged her marriage. That done, the young man waited for the girl. When she brought in the cattle, her intended and his friends forced her to go with them. Regardless of whether she liked the young man or not, she fought with her hands and feet, nails and teeth. She was dragged kicking and screaming to her father's tent, and a man's cloak was thrown over her. She was changed into clothes supplied by her husband-to-be and flung, still struggling, onto a camel.

She was taken to the young man's tent, still fighting, and there the young man had intercourse with her, she still resisting whether she wanted the man as a husband or not. The next morning, if she was agreeable, she stayed with her man. If not, she was returned to her father. A woman taken in this way who was either divorced or a widow was considered bad-mannered if she struggled in the manner of a virgin.

The Arandan girl of central Australia was abducted when she came of marriageable age. Male relatives of her intended, as well as other marriageable young men, seized her and took her into the bush. They took her virginity with a knife, then had gang sex with her, painted her, dressed her up and delivered her to her intended.

Interbreeding and incest have had their place in history:

Because the ancient Greeks followed the family through the mother's line, a man was forbidden to marry his half-sister born to his mother. It was considered incestuous. However, since his lineage on his father's side was of no importance, he could marry his half-sister by his father, with no trouble.

The northern Japanese Ainu man could not marry his mother, his sister or his sister-in-law, but he was allowed to marry his cousin, niece or daughter.

The mothers of Aleut boys often married their sons.

The central Borneo tribe of Murungs viewed marriage between cousins as a horrible sin, but allowed brothers and sisters to marry.

In British New Guinea, on the island of Kiwai, marriage between brothers and sisters was regarded with revulsion, but fathers and their daughters frequently married.

Among the ancient Incas of Peru, the eldest sister in a family married her brother.

Interbreeding and incest have had their place in history:

In most parts of the world, incest has been strictly taboo. It was most vigorously opposed through the customs of marriage:

In the Burmese villages of the Zayeins, the single men and women lived separately in large huts at opposite ends of the villages. The two sexes were kept segregated and were so apprehensive toward each other, they did not look each other in the eye. Part of the reason for this shame and fear was the penalty for interaction with a member of the opposite sex of the village: The offenders were killed after digging their own graves. Sexual relations and marriage between persons of the same village was considered the most horrible kind of incest.

While not apparently sexually incestuous, the marriage contract has produced intimacy between brothers and sisters-in-law:

Young southern Slav and Balkan Peninsula women had the groom's brothers as bridal attendants. They became very intimate with the groom's brothers. By custom, however, they were not permitted to be as open with their husbands as with the brothers-in-law. They did not speak to their husbands in public and were bashful around them in private. On the other hand, they kept their brothers-in-law as close confidantes—their only close friends.

The most common form of allowable incestuous relationship has been the sharing of a sister-in-law:

In Tibet, several brothers often shared the same wife, she having marital relations with as many as five brothers.

A Gilbert Islander, when attracted to one girl, married all her sisters as well. This was mainly for economic reasons, because each daughter had an equal share in her father's estate.

In ancient Britain, husbands had 10 or 12 wives. These wives were shared with other men, especially between brothers. In some cases, father and son practiced this kind of partnership.

Among the ancient Chinese, the concept of marriage was a union not just between two people, but between families. This sense of community was so strong that the marital connection that had been pre-arranged was almost always kept—even if one or both of the partners to be married were dead and buried.

Incest has taken the form of custom—and duty:

In East Africa, both the Wahele and the Wagogo tribes practiced ritual incest. Before being allowed to marry his sweetheart, the young man was required to sleep with his mother-in-law.

Being married, throughout history and around the world, has taken on very many different meanings:

Ancient Islamic law had a liberal form of marriage. Citizens in that region could enter into Muta, or marriage for only a certain limited length of time.

The ancient Romans had a form of trial marriage called Usus. A couple were considered permanently married if they lived together continuously. This trial marriage was dissolved if the man and wife separated themselves from each other for three straight days and nights. The one-year trial period started again after they returned to each other.

Women unsure of the prospective husband's qualifications, or merely wishing to be treated better than the married woman was, regularly separated themselves from their live-in mates. With properly timed absences from her "husband," a woman could prolong the period of courtship indefinitely.

In the mid-1700s the residents of South Wales, particularly miners, were married in their own manner. Whether they did not want to pay the church the marriage fee, or they considered the formalism impractical, they chose to marry in a most convenient way. They called this alternate wedding Priodas, or "Little Wedding." To share the expense of a civil ceremony (cost: three mugs of ale), a handful of couples would be married at once. Often they even shared the same honeymoon accommodations.

The Little Wedding could be broken by either party, but it was usually terminated by the miner who relocated because of his work. A woman who had been married in this way but was no longer, lost none of her honor in having been temporarily married.

In ancient Scotland, a couple could marry simply by announcing themselves so in front of witnesses. It was common for English couples eloping to choose this route. A Scottish village famous for receiving English elopers was Gretna Green. The blacksmith shop was the sight of very many hasty weddings.

The man who performed many of the weddings was not a clergyman, but a landlord, David Laing. When he retired, his son, Simon, performed the ceremony. Another resident, Robert Elliot, married approximately 4,000 couples from 1811 to 1839.

For three-quarters of the Christian era, it was most common to marry without a holy man officiating. The marriage was considered completely legal. It was not until 1563, the year of the Council of Trent, that a couple were required to marry with ceremony and witnesses.

Among many primitive tribes, a man and a woman were united when they ate rice out of the same bowl.

The wedding ceremony of the Nairs of Cochin, Malabar and Travancore had a meaning very different from most marriage ceremonies. Before a girl reached womanhood, she was married to a stranger. A marriage collar was placed around her neck and the couple completed the occasion by going to bed together.

The "husband" stayed three days, divorced the girl, received a fee and left. The girl went back to her family, and only after the night spent with the man started seriously considering possible husbands. At this time, she kept house with many lovers. The man who slept with her for a fee was the only man she could not consider as a husband. She then accumulated from 4 to 12 husbands.

The Haidan Indian of the Americas practiced trial marriage. In this west coast tribe, a boy took a wife for a month. If she was satisfactory, she stayed. If she displeased him in any way, she was returned to her family, no questions asked.

⚥

While almost all cultures have viewed romance and affection as desirable features of marriage, some have had no use for it:

The Mehinaku Indians, inhabitants of the Tuatuari River on the Amazon River system, viewed romanticism with scorn.

There was little real affection shown between lovers, and any demonstration of tenderness was very slight. New lovers were permitted a small amount of freedom to express their attachment, but public display of affection between husband and wife was considered to be in very poor taste.

⚥

Once married, ancient couples had the duty and responsibility of increasing the race. Given the importance of this function to the society, there was much discussion and advice on the subject:

In Deuteronomy 24:5, in the King James version of the Bible, men were instructed to give their undistracted sexual attentions to their wives. It suggested that new husbands be exempt from military service: "When a man hath taken a new wife, he shall not go out to war, neither shall be charged with any business; but he shall be free at home one year, and shall cheer up his wife [who had to leave her parents] which he hath taken."

At one time, it was thought that the female had a higher sex drive than the male. In II Samuel 6:20-23, it was suggested that a man could punish his wife by withholding his sexual advances to her. Women's

151

desires were to be distrusted so much that there were severe limitations placed on the meeting of men and women.

The Jewish husband could not, because of a dispute, be absent from his wife on a weekend; if he did so, she could sue him.

The Indian Arthasastra of Kautilya declared that a husband should pay a fine of 96 panas if he did not have intercourse right after her period stopped.

Life after marriage could very often fall far short of married bliss:

In China, the groom did not see his bride until the procession brought her to his home. He then opened the door to her sedan and saw her for the first time. If he was disappointed, he immediately closed the door of the sedan and sent her home—the wedding, in full swing, called off.

The Masai groom of East Africa was obligated for a full month after his wedding to wear his wife's clothes.

In some African tribes, the wives of a chief served as furniture. The wives rivaled each other for the chance to be used by their husbands as chairs, pillows and stools.

A new groom in the Khasis tribe moved into his wife's parents' home. He was treated very poorly, being called shong kha, or begetter. He was treated like a stranger. If the couple's stay was a success, they set up their own household after the birth of a child or two.

Butan women were required to carry their husbands on their backs when traveling.

An unusual living arrangement existed among the Maoshai and Syntengs. Husband and wife did not live together. The extent of their relationship was in his visits to her.

In British New Guinean Moto, the husband left his wife and his hut to sleep in a hut with the rest of the married men of the village, as was their custom. This provided the wife the opportunity to sample the talents of the single men of the village. She very often entertained young bachelors while her husband was away.

The Kansas and Osage Indian tribes were matriarchal. Once the eldest daughter married, the power of the household switched from the daughter's parents, especially her mother, to the eldest daughter. The newly married eldest had control in all affairs. Younger sisters became wives of their sister's husband.

The rights and obligations given uncles over their nieces and nephews has been most common in South America and Africa:

Among the Goajiros of Columbia, a girl was given away in marriage by her uncle on her mother's side. The maternal uncle decided who she married. He also set the dowry, and when it was paid, the dowry was paid to the uncle—his to keep.

Brides have been asked to sacrifice some of their sexual charm in return for the comforts of marriage:

A very common practice among the ancients was cutting a new bride's hair off. Her hair being one of the woman's main attractions, it was removed so that she would be less alluring to other men.

Marriage, while offering the security of a helpmate, has also enslaved spouses:

The women of Loango were allowed to speak to their husbands only while on their knees.

Aboriginal tribes often had limitations, rather than freedoms, as reward for having married the daughter of a family:

The man who married in the Poulh Indian tribe observed a strange custom. He was not allowed, from the time of his wedding, to look at his mother-in-law.

Nearly every culture in the world was protective of its newly married women:

The southern India Khonds had a custom whereby the brother of the bride's father, her maternal uncle, carried her from the ceremony to her new home on his shoulders. If he set her down before she got home, he was fined one buffalo.

It was unforgivable for the French bride of the early 1800s to be seen in public without being chaperoned by either her husband, mother or mother-in-law, for a full year after marriage.

Marriage has been responsible for the rapid increase in the size of a tribe or village. The prosperity of having many warriors or food gatherers has made almost all societies outlaw unions that were not productive in this way:

If an ancient Hebrew woman did not bear any children after 10 years of marriage, the husband was forced to divorce her, so that he could find a wife who could bear him children.

In societies' attempts to keep the family unit together, a legal form of adultery was allowed. This was permitted in the name of propagation:

In ancient India, a man who found himself unable to reproduce, either through impotence or sterility, hired a stand-in. This substitute was asked only to perform the reproductive act, then depart. The marriage between the two partners was unaffected by the sexual intimacy with the stranger.

The sterile or impotent man in Manu asked another man to lay with his wife. Once delivered, the child from the union was lawfully the husband's because the wife bore the child: "The seed and the fruits thereof belong lawfully to the owner of the field, no matter by whom the plowing was done."

The Bushongo bride, immediately following marriage, had intercourse with as many men as she could find, to become pregnant as soon as possible. This would provide her with children and quickly prove to her husband that she was a good (fertile) wife.

The powerful need and desire for children could be a very effective method to control behavior:

If the Damaras woman swore at her husband, she was never allowed to have sex with him again. For his part, he was not allowed, under any circumstances, to approach her for intercourse.

The East African Baganda husbands were very careful not to allow their wives to have affairs. There was the chance that she might have another man's child. As well, the husband whose wife stepped out on him was fined for not guarding her honor—while the wife and her lover were not punished at all.

The societal promotion of large families worked so well that even sophisticated societies, with relatively no direct economic need for large numbers, kept expanding quickly:

Before the Plague of 1710 in England, Lord Kames reported that the average English family had between 15 and 20 children. Given the strains which childbearing produced on the body, the average woman likely had several miscarriages as well, as in the case of a woman who had produced 14 children and had six miscarriages.

A great number of primitive societies had a mother-in-law taboo, which restricted relations between the son-in-law and his new relative:

In Northern Australia in certain tribes, the mother-in-law blew a horn in announcing her presence to her son-in-law. This provided him time to hide himself.

In southeastern Australia, the penalty for talking to one's mother-in-law was death.

The Catholic Church allowed very few circumstances that justified divorce. But one of them was sexual:

Pope Innocent III, during his reign (1198–1216), declared that a marriage could be dissolved when the genitals of a husband and wife did not manage to fit properly. If the difference in size of the genitals made it dangerous or impossible to have intercourse, the marriage was nullified.

The pain and humiliation people have endured to be true to public morality is nowhere better shown than in the 16th and 17th centuries:

A law initiated in the mid-1500s in France lasted over 125 years, even though it was extremely unpopular. This law was Congres. It was created to test the claims of couples who wished to dissolve marriages because of the fact that the marriage was not consummated, or that no children could come of the union, for whatever reason.

A couple who wished to dissolve the marriage on these sexual grounds was forced to take an oath to indulge in intercourse honestly and vigorously. Then, with surgeons and matrons looking on, the couple had to attempt intercourse.

While position has had its privileges, it also has had its responsibilities:

The practice of young couples eloping was not uncommon in Samoa. But it was highly irregular for the daughters of chiefs to elope. If she tried to elope or was seen after she eloped, she was beaten, and her hair was shaved off. Even if they had legalized the attachment by marriage, and even if they had children, they were still regarded with some disdain. The structure of pairing off had been broken; the villagers did not appreciate this breach of the rules.

In some instances, a girl never left the influence of her home, but seemed to be merely lent out:

In ancient Greece, the Athenian girl, once married, became a part of her husband's family. But she was still under the authority of her father. For whatever reason, her father could take her away from her husband and take her back home. He also had the right to marry her off to another man.

The husband of ancient Greece could divorce his wife on practically any grounds. However, once he had divorced, he could not marry a woman younger than his ex-wife.

Although marriage was widely promoted, divorce was often extremely easy to justify:

Hillel was a Babylonian doctor of Jewish law who lived from 60 B.C. to A.D. 10. Hillel believed that a man was entitled to divorce his wife for whatever reason he saw fit. Some of these grounds could include the man's infatuation with another woman, or the fact that the husband didn't like his wife's cooking.

Among the Gypsies, a divorce ceremony involved a sacrifice. A horse was let loose to run. Its behavior indicated the degree of the wife's fault in the divorce. The horse was then brought to the officiating priest and accused of the woman's crime. Then the priest stabbed the horse in the heart. The husband and the wife were divorced while standing on either side of the dying horse.

By Babylonian law, a husband usually divorced his wife for being unable to bear children. However, he could also divorce her, or, if he preferred, make her a slave, for simply spending too much money.

The Mandja woman could not be divorced because she had committed adultery; however, she could be divorced for being a poor cook or messy housekeeper.

The New Caledonian woman who was once the wife of a chief could never marry again. After her term with the chief, she was obligated to become a prostitute. A husband could not divorce his wife if she had slept with another man. She could be divorced, however, if she had no common sense.

The North American Navajo Indians had a very liberated outlook toward wives. They considered it the right of the woman to leave her husband if at all dissatisfied. They made provisions for the embarrassed male. To avenge the humiliation, the husband was entitled to kill someone.

⚥

In medieval England, in the county of Essex, the community gave a prize to the couple who did not voice any unhappiness with their married state after one year and one day of marriage. The custom was initiated by Lady Juga. In 400 years, only five couples applied for the award.

In later ages, the reward was also offered to the man who could honestly say that he had not regretted his marriage after one year and one day. In one area, the rule was that "he that repenteth not of his marriage in a year and a day, either sleeping or waking, may lawfully go to Dunmow and fetch a gammon [side] of bacon."

One writer claimed that in the 100 years of that custom, a mere two men had been able to collect the prize; one was a sailor who'd been gone to sea for most of the period, the other was married to a woman who couldn't speak.

⚥

In Chaldea, the newly married couple had the priest start a new fire in the house's fireplace. The fire, from then on, was to be kept forever burning. If the fire went out, for whatever reason, the couple was forced to divorce.

⚥

The Naga men of the Bengal Hills did not marry until they had "retired" from the active life.

⚥

Some societies removed widows or allowed them to withdraw themselves. They were perhaps seen as unproductive and a liability to the community:

The Arawak widow whose children were married joined a community of solitary widows. These women provided completely for themselves, and men were not a part of the community.

157

The South African widow in the Cape of Good Hope who remarried presented her husband with a gift. When her previous husband died, she was obliged to cut off a finger at the joint to indicate that she was not a virgin. On her wedding day, she presented this finger and joint to her new husband.

In ancient India, it was common for women to get rid of their husbands by poisoning them. It became such a problem that the ritual of the Suttee was adopted. A woman whose husband died was obligated to crawl onto his funeral pyre and be cremated alive.

Societal stability was ensured when a widow was assured of another husband:

Among the ancient Arabs, a woman whose husband died was obliged to marry one of his other wife's sons.

A number of cultures have made provision for the quick remarriage of a widower:

In the Sudan, a widower was offered his wife's sister, with the dowry required of him being smaller than if he were marrying into the family for the first time.

The British Columbian Shushwap widower, during the required mourning period, was held prisoner by the dead woman's family. He was released only on the condition that he marry their daughter, the dead woman's sister.

Remarriage of widows and widowers was approached with some caution in many parts of the world:

Should an Indian man from Punjab have wished to remarry for the third time, certain precautions were taken. To make sure that his third wife didn't suffer the same fate as his previous two dead wives, a ceremony was performed. To confuse the gods, the widower was married to a tree, bush or sheep dressed as a bride. This protected his new wife from the misfortunes of his previous wives.

The Wabemba man in the Congo whose wife died could marry her sister. Should the sisters have been married, there was only one solution. The husband of one of the sisters (his brother-in-law) allowed the widower to sleep with his wife for two nights. This done, he could now remarry outside the wife's family.

Some cultures have married off their dead:

The southern Sudan man of the Nuer tribe who died a bachelor, or who died without leaving sons, had his "soul" married off. To accomplish this, a man from the dead man's clan married a girl under his dead friend's name. The man had full rights and responsibilities as a husband to the woman.

Mates have been fondly remembered for the sexual gratification they bestowed on their partners:

Widows in Gippsland, Australia and Tasmania were often inclined to wear their dead husband's penises around their necks.

It is rare that a spouse terminates marriage other than through divorce, but it does occur:

The wives of the King of the Shilluks "divorced" him when he could no longer perform intercourse. Their method of divorce: strangulation at their hands.

When a widowed woman in Surinam decided to marry, she had to go through a ritual before taking a new husband. Before her marriage, she had to go to bed with a male from her dead husband's family.

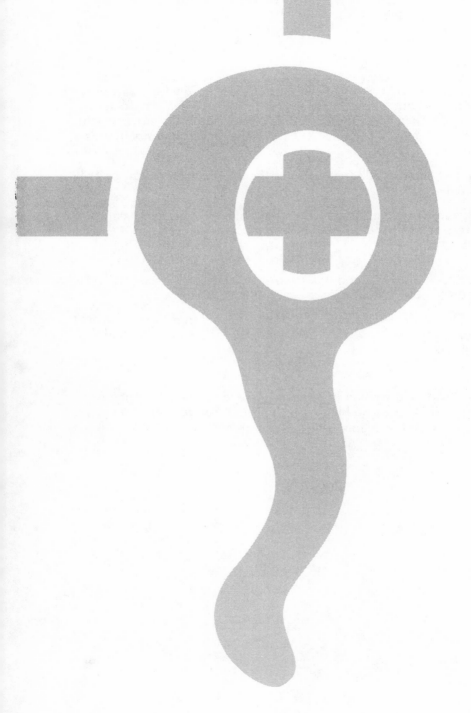

The Marriage Night

Among the nomadic Persians, a woman brought from her parents' home to her husband's home was met on her way by her husband. He carried with him either an apple or an orange. As she approached him, with all his might he heaved the fruit at her. The harder she was hit, the better her luck.

A new bride, now the property of a man, was jealously guarded:

To protect her modesty and honor, the Melanesian bride was transported to her husband's home by piggyback, with palm leaves covering her face and mats wrapped around her body.

A girl who kept her virginity was, in many societies, highly regarded:

In medieval France, on her wedding day, a bride was given a gift for keeping her maidenhead: a white hen, symbolizing her virginity.

In medieval Islam, virginity was highly prized in a bride: "O you who are giving away the girl after she has been deflowered, You are seasoning the pot after it has been overturned."

Sex has inevitably been a large consideration in marriage:

Among the heathen Anglo-Saxons, the woman's marriage vow included a reference to the sexual obligation: "I take thee to be my wedded husband, to have and to hold, from this day forward, for better for worse, for richer for poorer, in sickness and health, to be my bonny and buxom, in bed and at board, till death do us part, and thereto I plight my troth."

The sacrifice of the woman's maidenhead was a source of great gratitude and romance:

The romance of the hymen was strong in the 17th century. In the words of 17th-century writers, the breaking of the hymen during first intercourse was a romantic turn of nature; the "flower of the maidenhead" was "plucked" and the virgin who allowed "master mole" to "burrow within" was deflowered.

Next to the wedding process itself, the most important part of a union was the consummation, more especially the breaking of the bride's hymen:

Vandalism was performed in the 17th and 18th centuries in England, Germany and Slovakian countries: To commemorate the breaking of the maidenhead, the young people went about breaking all the old pottery in the bride's household.

The length of the marriage night has been variable. Some cultures promoted delaying the marital sex relation, while others celebrated this new life for a lengthy period:

The bride and groom of Flores Island, in the Malay Archipelago, spent their wedding night and three nights afterward with company. For these four nights they were watched by eight married women, who saw to it that the couple did not have intercourse.

The marriage night for the Urubu tribe of Brazil actually lasted 10 days. The husband and wife closeted themselves, making love continuously, only stopping to regain their strength and sexual powers.

Most rituals of the marriage night were public displays. There have been few private rituals performed on the first night as husband and wife:

Among the Russians, part of the formality of going to bed for the first time as husband and wife was the very intimate act of removing each other's stockings. This represented their sexual commitment to each other.

Throughout the world, the dowry represented the price of a bride's virginity:

Among the Welsh in the Middle Ages, a husband paid his wife a dowry for her virginity, an Agweddi, after they had performed their first intercourse.

Sometimes marriage was the product of intercourse, rather than intercourse being the result of marriage:

Among the Samoans, a couple usually had intercourse before they were considered married. The young man proposed, and the union was confirmed by spending the night and making love at her parents' hut. It was only by having intercourse that they were considered husband and wife.

The sacrifice of the woman's virginity was not always through intercourse:

In ninth-century Japan, a bride-to-be was escorted the night before her wedding to the Ise shrine. In front of the sun goddess Amaterasu, the girl's virginity was taken by a wooden phallus, or sometimes by the priest himself.

In ancient Rome, the role of deflowering the bride was publicly given to a sculpture of the god of fertility. The new bride lowered herself on the ever-erect stone phallus of Mutunus Tutunus, and in this way was blessed with many children.

The Jatt bride of Baluchistan, before she had intercourse with her new husband, admitted an old lady into the marriage chamber. The old lady took out a razor and "deflowered" the girl. The new bride was then expected to have her first marital intercourse.

To assure that the marital obligation was carried out, there were often designated witnesses whose right it was to observe the embrace:

A Tongan bride took a very old female relative to the marriage bed with her and her new husband. The old woman witnessed their intercourse. Should the old lady have known or suspected that the girl had already lost her virginity, she protected the girl's pride and reputation. To do this, she stained the bed with the blood of an animal, satisfying both the groom and the relatives.

After the ancient Hebrew couple were married, they retreated to the couple's house with 10 of their male relatives. There, all prayed and then feasted. Eventually, two of the groomsmen took the bride and groom to the bedchamber. There, as witnesses, the two men observed the couple's first sexual embrace.

When an African Bakitara girl got married, her aunt was a close witness. The aunt went with her to her niece's new home. There, she witnessed the couple's first married night. If the girl was hesitant, her aunt instructed her during the lovemaking. If the girl was shy, the aunt often took the bride's place with the husband, to demonstrate.

The importance attached to virginity has made it necessary for the parents of a "fallen woman" to reclaim her virginity. This sham was widely accepted:

In ancient Persia, virginity was highly valued. But a girl who lost her maidenhead before marriage was often married off to a man of low status. Upon the marriage he signed a certificate of virginity. It indicated that her virginity had been taken honestly by the husband himself. She would then divorce him, seeking a richer husband, and having cleared herself of shame.

Many societies have been careful to observe the loss of a new wife's virginity. Her purity was an absolute requisite for marriage, so there were many customs to observe that the girl was properly deflowered:

The Bedaui villagers were given absolute proof of a girl's honor. On her wedding day, a woman took the bedcover with the stain of her virginity on it, and placed it on a spear in the middle of the village for all to see.

In parts of ancient Peru, the bride's mother deflowered her daughter. With the groom's relatives looking on, the mother used her fingers to break her daughter's hymen. By doing this, the mother showed pride and confidence in her daughter's purity. The ceremony was proof to the in-laws that the girl had been brought up properly.

The daughter of a Samoan head chief, or Taupo, did not lose her virginity in the privacy of her parents' hut, as commoners did. On the marriage day, in a brightly lit hut in front of everybody, the tribe's talking-chief took the young bride's virginity.

In parts of India, after the wedding ceremony, the bride, groom and their families and guests retreated to the bridal house. While the others visited, the bride and groom retired to the bedroom. Family and friends waited to hear the bride's cry as she lost her virginity. The guests waited quietly, because it was a bad sign if it was not heard by all. The groom did his best to make his wife heard by penetrating her as violently and painfully as possible. Once the yell was heard, a priest broke a coconut over a red stone which resembled a penis. This ritual celebrated the loss of virginity.

A Turkish woman who married but wasn't a virgin could expect her new husband to make love to her for three nights in a row. The virgin's husband, however, was obligated to make love to her for seven straight nights.

For a very long time in history among the civilized peoples, it was no shame for friends and relatives to want the bridal couple to "share" their wedding night:

Among the Burmese, on the wedding night young men crowded around the home of the newlyweds, armed with rocks and other objects. Through the night they threw these objects on the roof and through the windows. Very often this exercise damaged the house badly, and it was not unusual that it resulted in injuring the couple trying to celebrate their marriage night.

It was a regular custom for 18th-century American residents in Rhode Island to involve themselves in the wedding night. Young men frequently good-naturedly kidnapped the bride from the bridal chamber and forced the groom to rescue her.

The French, as recently as the Renaissance, made the wedding night something of a public spectacle. Guests shared the wedding night with the bride and groom by trying to view the performance from outside the windows of the bedchamber and listening at the door. Some tried to peek into the room through the door or climb up to the bedroom window. The bride's screams and groans, and the "moving of the straw," or creaking of the bed, provided voyeurs with reason to cheer and applaud the groom's efforts.

In the south of Sweden, it was common until the 18th century that the bridal couple undressed for bed in front of the wedding guests.

The ancient Chinese had a tradition called Warming Up the Wedding Chamber. Wedding guests hurried through the banquet in anticipation of joining the bride and groom in their wedding chamber. The "warming" consisted of embarrassing attempts at making the bridal couple blush.

Guests told dirty jokes and demanded that the bride do the same. They cheered and persuaded the bride and groom to "drink from the flesh cup." This was the passing of a mouthful of wine from the groom's to the bride's mouth. If any wine was spilled in the transfer, they were obliged to try again.

The crowd's pleasure was to see the bride in total and utter embarrassment. One of the more popular chamber games was called Touching the Fish. In it, the humiliated groom was forced to put his hand into the bride's garment and give a description of his discoveries within.

Very often, if the bride was attractive, the guests teased the couple for several hours. By tradition, they were entitled to tease the bride for three consecutive nights.

(é

A nervous couple could not always afford the luxury of practice in the marital relation:

Tancredus (1185–1236) advocated that a new husband should have only three chances at deflowering his bride. If he could not do so after the three strikes, Tancredus advocated that the marriage should be dissolved.

(é

The wedding night was not always a romantic, intimate affair:

A sultan often rewarded a courtier by giving him his daughter in marriage. However, being a princess, she had ultimate control over him, as the wedding night proved. She was installed on a sofa, and he entered, bowing. He bowed again halfway to her, then again at her feet. He proclaimed his love for her and his high hopes of making her happy.

She drew a dagger, threatening him, and he quickly countered by pulling out the sultan's decree of their marriage. She withheld the dagger and said, "The sultan's will be done," and accepted the man as her husband.

(é

The pressure of performance led some couples to believe they might be cursed:

It is not clear how common a practice it was, but in Renaissance France, it was documented that an officer from the ecclesiastical court exorcised evil spirits from a couple who had trouble consummating their marriage. The officer, from the court of Chateaudun, took the pair to a garret, tied each facing the other to a post, and persistently whipped them with a birch rod. He then untied them and left them for the night with the door locked. By morning, the couple had been successful in their first intimacy.

(é

The deflowering of the bride, in some cases, could take a long time to occur:

The King of Tamassii left the defloration of a virgin wife to the first stranger who entered the village following her marriage.

At other times, formal deflowering of the bride took place well before marriage:

A girl on the island of Mitylene was given to a stranger passing through. If the man was of some status, he could choose his partner from the available girls. If not, he was assigned a girl. The two were "married," and the marriage feast held. The couple celebrated the wedding night. The next morning the stranger was required to leave. The girl would then marry a Myletenian a year after her "marriage." Losing her virginity to a stranger was a happy occasion for the girl; to lose her virginity to a Myletenian was considered an embarrassment to the local girls.

For the most part, the consummation of a marriage has taken place in at least relative privacy. There have been exceptions:

Some ancient Greek philosophers, called Cynics, believed that what was good and right could be spoken of and seen by all. Some Cynics, such as Crates and Hipparchia, went so far as to apply this concept to the wedding night, when they made love in front of their guests.

A Namaqua couple experienced their first married sex while their marriage feast was going on, in full view of all the guests.

It has happened that the new husband spent more of his wedding night watching than participating:

The Banaro lived on the banks of the Ceram River in New Guinea. Weddings were held in groups of four, each woman marrying a boy from another clan. Nine months before the wedding, they were led to a hut and lived there. The morning of the wedding, they were released; as they left, they were greeted by a hailstorm of coconuts and driven into a river.

Afterward they were dressed for the wedding dance. In the evening, when it came time for the consummation of the marriages, the groom's fathers expected to deflower the daughter-in-law. They protested and claimed to be too ashamed; instead, a friend within the father-in-law's clan did it. After he'd had sex with the bride, the friend then took the girl back to her mother's house. The bridegroom's father then took the virginity of his clan friend's son's wife. The groom was not allowed to have intercourse with his bride until a child was born to her.

Southern Malabar's King of Calicut followed the tradition of his

ancestors. Since the maidenhead was considered a nuisance to the pleasures of sex, he employed the High Priest to rid his wives of their virginity. As reward for this chore, the High Priest was paid 500 crowns
per performance.

This custom, when adopted by the common people of southern
Malabar, was bastardized. The blessing of the High Priest, and his role in
merely ridding the girl of her hymen, was misinterpreted. Consequently,
the point behind the role of the High Priest was mistaken.

The people of southern Malabar, not realizing the reason behind the
custom of the defloration by the High Priest, took this exercise a step
further. They believed in the groom's lack of qualification for deflowering his new wife. Brides instead gave themselves to the wedding guests—
the senior men first.

In ancient Phoenicia, the new bride was deflowered by a wooden phallus the day before her wedding. She then had sex with every unmarried
man in the village.

A number of cultures have recognized gang-sex as the ideal introduction of a bride into the marital relation:

Some Turkish peoples had a custom until the 20th century that
involved the Melauzim. Melauzim was the custom of the groom offering his bride to his friends, before taking his own pleasure. In one
19th-century incident, a young man enlisted in the army honored the
custom. The bride entertained his whole regiment, 100 men, on the
wedding night. Privates were entitled to one orgasm, officers, several.
The young husband's colonel, appreciating the man's regimental loyalty, promoted the groom to the rank of captain.

The privilege of taking the fruits of a woman's innocence has often been
a matter of power, not possession. It could be stolen from a husband:

The East Indian Somorin man did not have first sexual possession of
his wife. That privilege belonged to the Nambourie, or chief priest,
who enjoyed the new bride for the first three nights of her marriage
before turning her over to her husband.

Jus Primae Noctis, or "Right of the first night," was likely an offshoot
of Culagium, the request for permission to marry. Since the landlord in
feudal times often lost a taxpayer when the woman moved from her
house to her husband's, he felt he was entitled to compensation. A
marchet (or merchet, marchetta or marquetta), a penalty, was paid to
reimburse the landlord.

This right was stated by a Lord in Bourdet, Normandy: "I have a
right to take from my men and others, when they marry on my lands,

10 sols tournois and a joint of pork, with a gallon of whatsoever drink is drunk at the wedding; and I may and ought, if it pleases me, go and lie with the bride, in case her husband or some person on his account fail to pay to me or my command one of the things above rehearsed."

Should the king decline the opportunity to bed the new bride, an underling could take his place; however, it was not without expense for the minor official. In this case, the law of Jus Primae Noctis was as such:

> The groom shall invite the manager of the estate to the wedding and he shall so invite the manager's wife. The manager shall bring a cartload of wood to the wedding, and the wife shall bring a quarter of a roasted pig. When the wedding is over, the groom shall let the manager [if the King transferred his right to the manager] lie with his wife the first night, or he shall redeem her with five shillings and six pence.

A medieval custom in England very commonly used was what amounted to a bribe. Traditionally, the Christian Church demanded that the newlyweds spend the first three nights of their marriage in chastity. However, a fine could be paid to the church in order that the husband and his bride could exercise the marital privilege. This allowed the couple to "sin" with the permission of the church's treasury.

Very often monks demanded the right to deflower new brides, if they were so inclined. This was the case in France in St. Auriol, during the Middle Ages. The monks of St. Thiodard frequently slept with the new brides.

The Mekeo girl of New Guinea slept with her new father-in-law for three weeks—and during this time her husband was not allowed to approach her sexually.

The wedding night was not always an assurance of pleasure and constant sexual satisfaction:

The ancient Greek essayist Plutarch (A.D. 50–120) reported a Spartan marital custom. A girl would cut her hair to look like that of a man. Then the husband-to-be symbolically abducted her from her parent's house.

She wore men's clothes for the abduction. The wedding night consisted of the husband eating at the mess hall with his friends, then coming to her and performing the first married intercourse with her. After the act, he returned to his barracks. This schedule was the extent of their married life until he was discharged from the army at the age of 30.

Many sexual customs must have severely tested the excitability of partners:

A Spartan bride prepared for her wedding night by dressing in male clothing. Then a female attendant shaved the girl's head. The bride then awaited the groom on the bridal bed.

In Cos in ancient Greece, the male greeted his wife on the wedding night wearing a dress.

The Tartar groom entered his bride's house very carefully, and the next morning took great care not to be seen leaving. If he were spotted by his new bride's relatives, he was customarily beaten severely by her family.

The East African Somal bride entered the bridal chamber fully expecting a painful greeting. Upon the woman's entrance, her new husband greeted her, whip in hand, and began the wedding night by whipping her.

Galla and Somali girls had their labia stitched together to assure their husbands that they were virgins at marriage. This practice was called infibulation. The Somali and Galla husbands did not break his infibulated bride's stitches with a knife, the way some lovers did. Instead, the groom increased his intake of meat before the wedding to increase his strength. On his wedding day, he forced the stitches open with an assault by his penis. This was painful for the bride and usually unsuccessful for the groom. Often he used his finger, or failing that, a knife to part the stitches. The pain usually made the bride cry out; male and female musicians sang and made noise to drown out the shrieks of pain. After the wedding night, the couple spent a week in their hut, making love continuously.

The Nubian girl, whose vaginal lips had been sealed together, only allowing a narrow opening for the passage of urine, was prepared for the marriage night. An aunt widened the tiny opening in the vagina by inserting a block of wood to stretch the opening. Then, on the wedding night, the aunt took a knife and cut the sealed lips open. Immediately after this, intercourse took place.

The sacrifice of the night before was often acknowledged the morning after:

The French had a custom, perhaps borrowed from the ancient English, of keeping lamps burning for four days after the wedding. During this time the bride stayed in bed day and night. She received well-wishers while in her bed. This was the sign that the wife, supposedly inexperienced, was quite exhausted, and that the husband had been so virile the first night of their lovemaking that she needed a long recovery time.

The Samoyed bride had to hide her face from her husband for two months after her marriage, only revealing her face when her husband had sex with her.

The sexual act, even within a marriage, has often been considered dirty, and has left a taint on the newly experienced couple:

A newly married couple in medieval England was not allowed to go to church for 30 days after the consummation of their marriage. They were also obligated to do 40 days' penance, and when returning to church, obliged to bring an offering.

The Roro New Guineans arranged marriages between villages to everyone's satisfaction. The wedding was occasion for a festive inter-village feast, enjoyed by all. However, the morning after the wedding night, it was the custom that the new father-in-law stood outside the couple's hut and verbally insulted and abused his new son-in-law. Then the bride's village attacked the groom's village, pretending to ransack the huts and gardens.

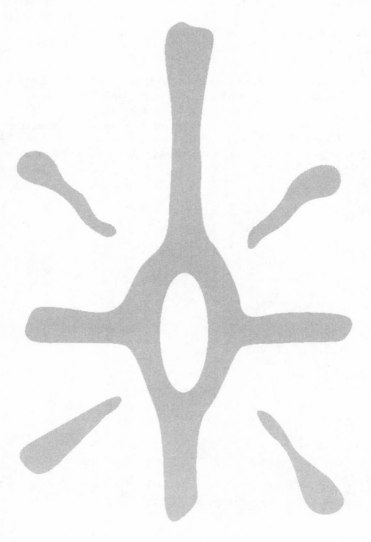

Birth Control

Birth control has been a subject of interest for many centuries. There have been many recipes to provide a couple with worry-free sex:

Aristotle, the Greek teacher-philosopher (384–322 B.C.), considered olive oil mixed with either cedar oil, lead ointment or frankincense to be the ideal contraceptive. This mixture was applied to "that part of the womb in which the seed falls."

An ancient Roman woman wishing to avoid pregnancy wore a leather pouch on her left foot during sex. In the pouch was a cat's liver.

One popular contraceptive in ancient Islam, up to at least the 13th century, was the use of elephant droppings inserted into the vagina.

The women of ancient Rome, to prevent having a child, were advised to spit into the mouth of a frog three times.

Exercises for the prevention of fertilization of the female have also been recommended:

Whores in first century B.C. Greece supposedly ground their pelvises in such a way as to increase their partner's pleasure. This practice was also believed to prevent pregnancy; the movement, they believed, diverted the sperm away from the womb.

Soranus of Ephesus was a gynecologist of the early second century. His approach to keeping the male from fertilizing the female:

> The woman ought, in the moment during coitus when the man ejaculates his seminal fluid, to hold her breath, and

173

draw her body back a little so that the semen cannot penetrate the mouth of the uterus, then immediately get up and sit down with bent knees, and in this position provoke sneezes.

✝

Anal sex has, for the most part, been taboo among the world's cultures. But this pleasure had its supporters:

The women of the Mohave tribe in New Mexico welcomed anal intercourse. It was a pleasure they knew would not result in pregnancy. For this reason, it was considered a favor by the male toward the female—showing kindness and consideration for the female.

✝

In 19th-century America, women of the Midwest tried to procure abortions by rubbing gunpowder over their breasts, or drinking tea consisting of rusty nail water.

✝

One of the most ingenious methods of birth control was invented by Australian natives, who were amazingly resourceful:

The aborigines of Australia practiced a surgical method of birth control. Called the Mika operation, it involved slitting the male's urethral canal. In this way, the semen was diverted sideways, away from the head of the penis and discharged outside the vagina.

✝

The beliefs of some cultures have been remarkably naive:

A ceremony performed before marriage by the African Hottentots was supposed to prevent the birth of twins: They cut the husband's right testicle off.

In some places, the moon was thought to be responsible for fertilizing the crops. For this reason, the women of these tribes took care to sleep out of the moonlight, for fear of being impregnated by moonbeams.

✝

The awareness of the sex–procreation relationship has usually spurred some sort of demand for birth control—though not always appropriate:

Papuan Islanders recognized the connection between sex and the bearing of children. Concerned that homosexual males might become pregnant, they devised a ceremony to avoid that possibility. Large public ceremonies were held to ensure that the catamites did not get pregnant. At this ceremony, the young men and boys were fed limes to assure contraception. The ritual proved very successful.

In 1532 Emperor Charles V forbade the use of birth control. The penalty for using contraceptives was death.

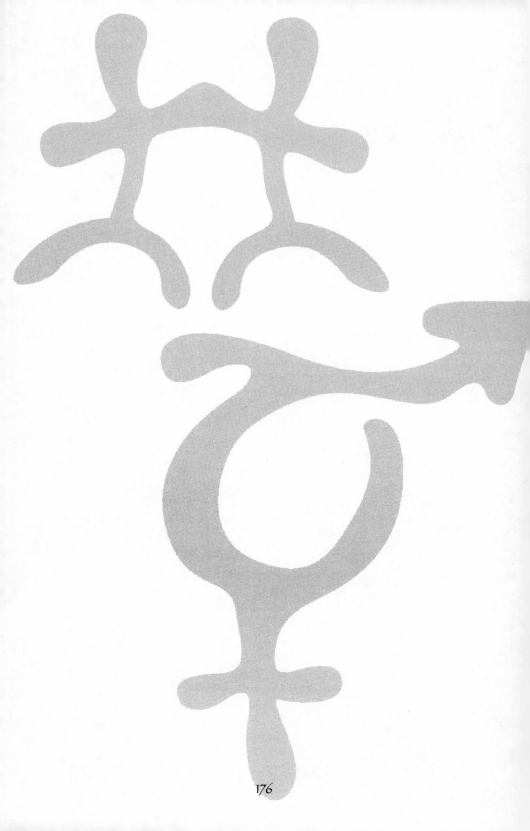

Beauty

Women have enlisted the help of the gods to make themselves desirable:

In early Roman-British Londinium, many street corners were adorned with Herms. The Herm was a square stone pillar about six feet tall, with a sculpture of the god Hermes on top. On one of the sides was carved a large erect penis and testicles. Women passing the Herm touched, stroked or kissed the stone phallus in hopes of becoming more sexually desirable.

※

Careful grooming has typically been associated with females. But some males have been equally fussy concerning their looks:

In preparation for a little nighttime carousing, Marquesan boys spent a great deal of time making themselves attractive. They bathed thoroughly, doused themselves in perfume and prepared their hair with a solution. Then, as a finishing touch, they pinned flowers behind their ears.

※

Sophisticated society often finds ancient culture to be most titillating:

Women of society in 19th-century Britain looked to the past to make themselves sexually alluring. The women of the upper classes followed the example of the ancient Egyptians and Italians, and had their nipples pierced. Through the holes pierced in their nipples, the women hung little gold rings.

Most beautifying procedures have accentuated youth. However, this has not always been the case:

The ancient Japanese woman used a mixture of nutgall in tannin with iron. Vinegar was added to this concoction. The product was then applied to the woman's teeth to make her more attractive. The result: It dyed her teeth black.

The northern Japanese Ainu girl tattooed her forehead, hands and arms. She also tattooed her upper lip. The bluish-black tattoo made the girl look very much like a man with a large mustache, stretching almost from ear to ear. This tattoo was usually completed by the groom when they took their honeymoon.

The bared breast was a feature of 17th-century costume in France—an outrage to the clergy of the time:

In the early 17th century, the fashion of exposing the breast was a source of disgust for moralists such as Father de Barry, who called the vanity of the breast a "plague-bearer and a venom which does empoison from afar when one casts one's eyes upon it, or when one touches it." Further,

> Breasts are not after all two small muck hills covered in snow, but two pounds of flesh which do cost a great deal to the foolish women who bare them and believe themselves thereby to be the more beautiful and the more pleasing. For their bosoms become cold from prolonged nudity, their swellings shrink down and do sometimes remain thus, when lo and behold death carries them off.

> A young lady of three-and-20 years did die of a sudden: the doctors had opened her up and could find no cause for her death other than a cold bosom. I have seen another die who was but seven or eight years old, but who had already been accustomed to having an uncovered breast.

The standards of beauty fluctuate between cultures and through time. Continually present, however, was the attraction of the earth-mother woman, whose large breasts and wide hips have represented nourishment and fertility:

The southern Cook Islands Mangaian man had a distinct preference for a woman with large hips. He believed that the woman's large hips provided her lover with more action, which allowed her to move better during sex. This more broadly built woman was referred to by the man as a 'bed with a mattress.'

Fashion has always played a large role in the sexuality of cultures. It has been used in many ways to achieve very different effects. From showing all to concealing all, fashion has titillated lovers for centuries:

In 1620 King James ordered the clergy to insist that women stop their lascivious fashion. He objected to the women wearing broad-brimmed hats as men did, wearing "wanton feathers," and cutting their hair like men in "ruffianly short locks."

In the Middle Ages, the church demanded the full enclosure of the female body to prevent lustful thoughts by men. As well, those parts of the female anatomy which aroused interest were to be cloaked. The bodice was introduced to reduce the curves of the female form. The bust was flattened and narrowed to make it inconspicuous. The female in the bodice took on an almost boyish look.

Little did the advocates of this style realize that many years later the bodice would inspire the corset. The construction of the corset was based on the bodice and made the bust look full and prominent. It also reduced the waist to as little as 13 inches around. This also emphasized the hips.

Seventeenth-century Spanish girls considered large breasts to be in poor fashion taste. For this reason, they wore heavy lead breastplates in order to stunt the growth of their breasts.

See-through clothing was worn as early as the ancient Greek and Roman eras. See-through togas were not unusual. Juvenal, the Roman satirist (A.D. 54–128) criticized judges for wearing transparent togas. Wearing these garments, he said, did not command much respect.

New Ireland native women were essentially naked until missionaries set up on the island. They provided the women with petticoats to cover their vaginas. The native women gratefully accepted the clothing. However, they would wear the petticoats only on their heads.

From the Middle Ages to the 17th century, the fashion among European women was the stomach. Dresses were padded over the abdomen to make the woman look pregnant. These artificial bellies were made of tin and called pads or paddies. Single women were especially fond of wearing these bloated-belly styles.

In the Middle Ages, men began to suggest something of their anatomy through their dress. An exaggeration of the male organ was the cod-piece. Originally, soldiers wore a sponge-lined metal cup to protect their private parts. It evolved into a steel-screen lined leather purse that hung between the legs. Civilians of the lower class began wearing leather sheaths. The upper class followed suit, making them much more gaudy and obvious, being made of silk, often with ribbons, gold and jewels.

A variation of the cod-piece was even more inviting to the female eye. Voyeurism reached its height in the 14th century, when Frenchmen wore underneath their breeches something called a braguette. Originally the working-class men wore a small bag between their legs for money and tobacco. In the middle of the 15th century, it was adopted by men of rank. Similar to a cod-piece, it did not imitate the manly bulge. The container, instead of imitating the organ, merely accentuated the owner's endowment. It, too, was decorated with ribbons, lace and jewels.

For four centuries men and women in France wore shoes *a la poulaine*. From the 12th to the 16th centuries, ordinary citizens wore these shoes, which symbolized the penis. Kings such as Charles V (in October 1367), priests, popes such as Pope Urban V (in 1635), and moralists railed against these obscene shoes as encouraging immorality.

During the time of Restoration England, the fashion for women was a large bosom. Since the dresses were low-cut, a woman found it difficult to pad her chest. Eventually an enterprising merchant introduced false breasts made of wax. A thin veil was worn over these very realistic waxy breasts.

Moruland women were naked except for a few leaves hanging off their hips. This skirt did not go all the way around their bodies; the leaves did not cover their vulvae, only their buttocks. For these women, and among some other African tribes, the exposure of the breasts or vulva was acceptable; but if their buttocks were exposed, the women had to fall down onto their backs to hide their bare backsides.

Men and women through the ages have tolerated some very unpleasant procedures in the name of fashion:

In ancient Greece, the Greek warriors, especially Spartans, practiced phimosis. Also practiced by athletes, artificial phimosis was thenarrowing of the orifice of the penis and extreme lengthening of the foreskin. To accomplish this, they wore clamps and locks made of metal.

One of the more painful beautification practices was footbinding:

During the Chinese Sung dynasty, around the early 10th century, a certain Li Yu built a lotus flower six feet tall for his love, Yao-niang. He bound his love's feet up so tightly that they resembled petals of the flower, and made her dance on the oversized model. Other ladies of the court saw the beauty of the bound feet and imitated Yao-niang's footbinding procedure. This tradition has lasted almost 1,000 years.

The practice of footbinding, very common among the Chinese and Japanese in the past, had a twofold purpose. Not only were the bound feet seen as more attractive for being petite, it was thought to have a more direct sexual effect. According to Morache, footbinding made the mons veneris, the outer vagina, smaller. Subsequently, it was claimed, the pubic area was made smaller and tighter.

Fashion has always been considered a large part of feminine charm. At times women were intent on using fashion to their greatest advantage, no matter what the cost:

By the time of the mid-18th century, England's industry was catering to a phenomenal hunger for luxurious fashion. The power of fashion and the desire to be fashionable were extremely strong.

Often, garments were so expensively priced for many of the women and girls that they took to less than honorable ways of earning the money for them. A yearlong investigation into prostitution and adultery of the time revealed that 60 percent of these sexual indiscretions were caused by women's desires to be finely dressed.

Central Australian men protected their penises by attaching beads or a shell to their pubic hair.

Female underwear was first worn by Oriental women. The garment made its way to Europe through Venice. Panties were first worn by prostitutes, and for this reason the underwear was considered an undesirable piece of clothing. There was much resistance to female underwear simply because it was commonly worn by the fashionable, trendsetting prostitutes.

Women started wearing underwear rather late in history:

The "inventor" of female underwear in Western society was Henri II of France's wife, Catherine de Medici. While horseback riding sidesaddle, her skirts were frequently blown upward by the wind. This offered the gentlemen of the court a glimpse of those parts of Catherine that were to be seen only by her husband.

So Catherine initiated the wearing of women's underwear by donning Calcons. Far from being pleased with her step toward modesty, the Renaissance moralists were outraged by the innovation. While the male critics were perfectly comfortable in their underwear, they were firmly against the wearing of "panties": Women should leave their buttocks uncovered under their skirts. They should not appropriate a masculine garment but leave their behinds nude as is suitable for their sex!

Nearly every part of the human body has been altered or adorned to be sexually enhanced in some way:

It was the habit of the French lady of the mid-1500s to apply an ointment to her genital area. The ointment encouraged the growth of her pubic hair. It was the desire of the French woman of that time to have extremely long pubic hair, so that it could be "curled like a Saracen's [Arab's] moustache." With this accomplished, the pubic bush was then decorated with colorful bows.

The beauty ideal has included every extreme of body type:

In some central African tribes, a woman with a large, hanging belly was considered the ideal beauty.

In many of the African tribes, the ideal female body type was boyish— with the line of her figure nearly straight up and down. One compared the figure of the ideal woman to be "like a ladder." But there was another qualification: She was much admired if she had "ears like an elephant."

In West Africa in the Assini region, very large nipples were considered attractive. The girls constantly worked the nipples to increase their size. To help in this cosmetic procedure, the girl encouraged the larvae of some insects to attack the nipple. As a certain substance on the insect irritated the skin, the constant aggravation enlarged the nipple.

Some African tribes regarded long, pendulous breasts as one of the primary aspects of beauty. To encourage the flattened, elongated breasts, cords were wrapped around the girls' chests. In some cases, their breasts hung down to the girls' knees. Some natives around the Cape of Good Hope had been observed throwing their breasts over their shoulders to feed the children on their backs.

The Venda girls of southwest coastal Africa between the ages of 10 and

12 began pulling on their labia to stretch them and make them look attractive. If they did not do this, they were severely criticized and called lazy. They were insulted if they did not have loose-hanging labia: "You are like a tree that lends no hold. Just a hole without anything."

Some fashions have been used to disguise sexual experience: In England during the Restoration, women could buy wigs called muggets, or, more properly, merkins. These wigs were worn on the genitals. They were worn when a woman's pubic hair fell out because of venereal disease.

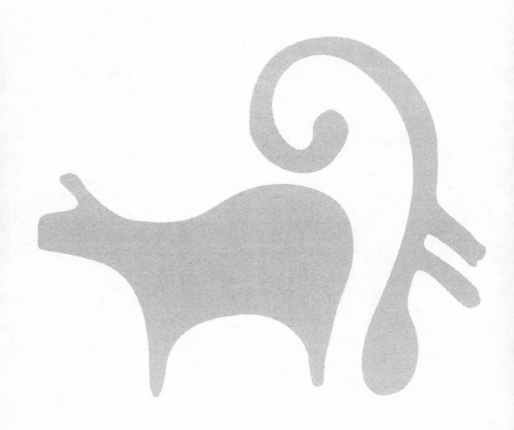

Pleasure

The 16th-century moral theologian Thomas Sanchez considered it a sin to have intercourse with a woman while she had her period. It was only allowable, he said, if it helped a marital crisis.

Tahitian women refused to perform fellatio on men, claiming that only "bad girls" engaged in it. However, cunnilingus was widely practiced. At the same time, both sexes considered kissing on the mouth a perversion.

Some public spectacles have had erotic overtones:

In the 19th century, public hangings were one of the most popular London amusements. The sadomasochism of these hangings drew crowds that some considered to be larger than any to be seen at any of the fairs or festivals of the day. Women were as keen to witness these executions as the males.

Often, young men and women entertained the executioners to extract all the grisly details of their experience. The morbid fascination with executions motivated citizens to walk as far as 20 miles to see the event, and pay high prices for the opportunity to view the spectacle from a window of a nearby building.

The hangings even provoked a "carnival of debauchery" among some communities. At Easton Road, a sale of hangman's ropes drew a huge crowd. The most popular ropes (especially where the ladies were concerned) were, predictably, those used to hang men who had committed crimes of passion and murdered their wives.

The instinct for life—and pleasure—has often been strongest at the time when man has seen death most closely:

During the syphilis epidemic of Middle Age Europe, the diseased victims of the ailment continued their sexual activities. Even the syphilitic sufferers in the hospitals kept having sex. Prostitutes were allowed to service patients who had even the most repulsive and advanced cases of syphilis.

Rape has primarily been a crime against females. There are exceptions:

The Melanesian Vakuta women felt perfectly entitled to rape men from other villages who may have strayed into their territory. They seized the man and, by acting lasciviously and masturbating him, induced erection. Then one woman mounted the male, inserting his penis into her vagina.

While she engaged in intercourse, the rest of the women urinated and defecated on their prisoner. His face was a favorite target. They also rubbed their genitals on his face and used his fingers to masturbate themselves.

A strict moral climate usually necessitated alternate methods by which citizens could exercise their amatory fantasies and desires:

The theater of the Middle Ages frequently masqueraded titillation under the guise of piety. Morality plays were performed that showed, in vivid detail, mistakes of human beings and their subsequent repentance. While characters were in the heathen state, the audience was treated to various scenes of nudity and obscene language.

One such play was the life of the whore Mary Magdalene, complete with highly realistic scenes of her life as a prostitute. Other plays featured characters representing the seven deadly sins, with suitably sinful behavior featured.

At certain times in history, the art of pleasure seeking was highly organized and even bureaucratic:

In ancient Rome, sexual indulgence was pursued in every way, in the Palace of the Caesars. These orgies were frequently hosted by the Roman noblemen's wives and daughters, and organized very efficiently by a government bureau of pleasure seekers called the Ministry of Pleasure.

The King of Dahomey had several thousand wives. He had intercourse with each once or twice; then they were obligated never to have sex again. Even though past her usefulness with the king, no man was allowed to look upon the king's wife. A servant walked in advance of the women and rang a bell or yelled for every man to leave the spot. Anyone at close distance was obligated to look away or fall face down on the ground.

For those who could afford it, sex could be supplemented with other pleasures of the senses:

During the Chinese Chou dynasty, aristocratic couples listened to music to set the tone for bedtime pursuits. Thereafter, lovers during later eras in the Imperial Palace chose to have the music accompany their sexual activities. The musicians played for the couple in the royal bedchamber as the couple went about their lovemaking.

The ancient Japanese shogun enjoyed complete privacy when he spent the night with one of his wives. But when he had a bout of lovemaking with a concubine, the couple shared the room with a female chaperone, called an ojoro. She had a bed, separated by a paper partition, on the other side of the shogun's bed. She was forbidden to fall asleep and had to file a report of the night's events the next morning. This eavesdropping ensured that the concubine did not ask for personal or political favors in return for her affections, and to ensure that should the concubine become pregnant, it was in fact by the shogun and not a lover.

In nearly all cultures, the male-female connection has been the ideal for pleasure. There have been some exceptions:

New Guinea's Marind-Anim men indulged in homosexual intercourse before marriage. The men were very fond of the practice and generally settled for marriage and heterosexual intercourse only when they absolutely had to.

The ability for a human male to see his partner's face during intercourse is unique among living creatures. Face-to-face sex is strictly a human act. However, many regions of the world have found this method unsatisfying and have preferred the way the animals practice it:

The most common position of intercourse among lovers in the Sudan was that of the woman standing, bent forward, hands on knees. Her partner approached her from the rear. This was also the preferred position for Eskimos and the Konjags.

The influence of the environment has had a profound effect on how humans showed their love:

The Kamchatkan people were primarily fish-eaters. Living on the coast, they took their cues from their environment. The Kamchatkan people refused to practice the woman-on-back, male-dominant position. They considered it sinful and believed in making love only by "imitating the fish." Both the male and female lay on their sides during the act.

Physical barriers to pleasure, even to the act of sex itself, have been the cause of much concern and sometimes laughter:

The Bushmen of the Kalahari Desert in Africa were often cruelly teased by neighboring tribes. The Bushman female had an unusually large mons pubis. Penetration with an erect penis was difficult, the penis having to be horizontal rather than vertical, to enter this type of vagina. Relations between the Bushmen and other tribes were always tense, because the other tribes made fun of the Bushman females.

On the Caroline Islands, a man inserted a piece of fish between his partner's labia and nibbled and sucked until the woman involuntarily urinated, due to sexual excitement. With this encouragement, he had intercourse with his lover.

The northern Japanese Ainu showed their affection not by kissing, but by biting. They bit the fingers, progressing up the arm and shoulders, then to the cheeks.

Among the New Guinea Mundugumor, a couple engaged in foreplay designed to be violent enough to excite the partners as quickly as possible. They vigorously bit and scratched to invigorate each other's passions. If the experience was particularly enjoyable, they tore off each other's jewelry and smashed it as a sign of their passion.

The central South American Chorowti women, during intercourse, expressed their pleasure and desire by spitting in their partner's faces.

It has been rare that the woman actively controlled the sexual act:

The Marquesans were one of the few peoples in which the woman controlled the sexual relationship. At feasts, which generally turned into orgies, the males sucked the females' breasts and performed cunnilingus. When the women felt prepared, they demanded intercourse.

The South Pacific Trukese woman insisted on sexual satisfaction. She laughed at the man who reached climax before she did, considering him a great failure, and insisted that he try again and do the job right.

Mankind has been diligent in overcoming the obstacles to sex and pleasure:

Ponape women were supposedly very frigid. They needed a great deal of stimulation to be aroused. Foreplay often lasted several hours. A couple usually employed an impotent old man to lick the woman's clitoris or sting it with an ant. This aroused and prepared the woman for sex.

Men have not always been the sexual aggressors. There have been instances when they have been the victims:

The Chinese aristocrats of the Manchu dynasty sought out every form of sexual thrill—or at least the men did. Soon frustrated at being ignored by their husbands and uninvited to the sexual revelry, the wives resorted to other methods. It was a frequent occurrence for a healthy young man to be kidnapped off the streets and taken to the anxious aristocratic wives for their sexual pleasure.

Among some tribes of the east central Carolines, during sex the man did not fondle his partner's breasts—instead he only rubbed his nose against them.

Baganda women of East Africa aroused their lovers to sex by tickling their men's armpits.

The East African Nandis were quite sexually modest. The husband and wife slept on separate sleeping mats a distance apart. A mound of earth divided the two beds. The male whispered endearments. When he cleared his throat, his partner knew he was ready for intercourse.

In a great number of societies, a woman who was rushed into sex without foreplay was insulted that she was being treated as a sex object, or that her readiness for sex was not considered. This attitude is not, however, universal:

The Mangaian man of the Cook Islands who attempted foreplay was usually treated with contempt. Mangaian women who agreed to have intercourse desired just that, and scorned the man who wasted her time with preliminary moves. Should a male linger too long without applying himself quickly to intercourse, he was referred to as a "limp penis."

The Baganda woman refused to cook for her husband if he did not have sex with her as often as she liked.

The East African Bagishu woman usually required that her husband satisfy her at least in the morning and again at night.

If he did not, she humiliated him into paying more sexual attention to her. She stood outside her hut loudly complaining for all to hear: "My husband's penis is dead!"

The Chiricahua woman of the American Southwest was not allowed to be sexually aggressive in the least. Not only could she not be aggressive, but during sex she was not allowed to show any emotion.

In Estonia, a husband was allowed whatever pleasure he wished with his wife. He was, however, forbidden to touch her breasts. It was thought that if he even brushed her breasts, her milk would be tainted when she later nursed a child.

The Tikopa of the Solomon Islands forbade the man to touch his genitals while sexually involved with his partner. She was not allowed to touch his penis, either.

The Annamites conducted intercourse in a unique way. The man did not wait for erection to occur before inserting his penis into his partner's vagina. The penis, half erect or even completely soft, was introduced into the vagina, and the woman constricted her vaginal muscles to massage the penis into erection.

Generally, the breasts and genitals of women have been the principal objects of sexual desire. There have been others, however:

Since the time of the Sung dynasty, Chinese eroticism has focused on feet—dainty, pointed feet. More than any other quality, feet were endowed with sexual allure. In erotic paintings, nude women with exposed vulvae were prominent—but their feet were always concealed.

The woman's feet were an important part of foreplay. While men could be forgiven for touching a woman's breasts or buttocks in a social situation, there was no excuse for any contact with her feet—that sort of intimacy was unforgivable.

The sexually skilled Chinese woman could offer the greatest erotic thrill desired by the Chinese man. These sexual experts were accomplished at giving their partners pleasure by playing with their partner's penises—with their feet.

Sexual customs have provided limited opportunity for sexual indulgence of some peoples:

The Druse were allowed to make love only once a month, after the woman finished her period.

In New Ireland, the husband and wife did not have intercourse while their pig was pregnant, and did not indulge until one month after it gave birth.

Wogeo women of northern New Guinea were considered to be cleansed of intercourse by menstruation. But men were required to cleanse themselves before intercourse as well. To protect themselves from disease as a result of intercourse, men periodically made incisions into their penises and allowed the blood to flow. About two months after this operation, once the cut had healed, the couple were allowed to have intercourse. If the man did not wait until the proper time, it was believed that both partners would die.

A large number of cultures have established appropriate periods of time during which new parents were not allowed to engage in sex. The lengths of time have varied—from token to lengthy:

In the New Guinea Highlands, the couples of the Dani tribe were required to abstain from sex from four to six years after the birth of their child. This practice was accepted and not considered a sexual hardship. It was not a problem for the couple, even though the Dani did not partake in any alternative sexual practices, such as homosexuality or masturbation.

Among some Caribbean peoples, the husband and wife did not have intercourse at night. This was because it was believed that if a child were created at night, it would surely be born blind.

The Gold Coast Tshi-speaking tribes had priestesses. These priestesses were not allowed to marry. But this did not prevent them from enjoying the pleasures of the flesh. In fact, they could have sex with any man they chose, and often had several lovers.

An ancient East Indian prayer indicated the proper time for intercourse: "At the time of the ritu do thou, O Lord of the Earth, approach thy wife happy under a constellation bearing a masculine name, at a propitious time, during the best even-numbered nights... nor near the holy trees...nor by cross roads, nor in places where many roads meet, nor in graveyards, nor in groves, nor in water...nor in twilight..."

Among many peoples, most commonly primitives, festive occasions featured unrestrained sex:

The faithful Zulu warrior could expect his chief to reward him periodically by way of Ukhlobonga. Ukhlobonga was the day when the unmarried women of the tribe provided several hours of ceremonial masturbation to warriors.

Ancient Roman women, showing contempt for the more sexually restrained life, mocked it. Some were said to have gone to the Temple of Chastity, and strapped an artificial phallus onto the goddess's statue. There, in turn, they took their pleasure on it.

Sadomasochism has found a steady clientele throughout the centuries, regardless of the moral climate and its restrictions toward the practice:

In the 18th century, flagellation became a favorite sexual activity in England. Whipping and beating was so popular in that age that brothels opened to deal exclusively with customers wishing to be sexually punished in this way.

The common people of 18th-century England were unashamedly open in their desire for sadomasochistic experience. An announcement of the schedule of activities for a Whitmonday, 1790: "A new hat will be the prize for men, a shift of Dutch linen for girls—in a drinking competition: further there will be a ball-game for a fine ham, a sack-race for a new pair of trousers, wrestling for a big plum pudding, and for a guinea—to get a sound thrashing."

The line between pleasure and pain has often been considered very fine:

The professional masseurs of 19th-century Berlin often had a sideline. In addition to working the flesh, these men often catered to the customer who desired to achieve orgasm in a dangerous but very intense way: The Berliner many times could buy the services of a masseur, who would hang the customer until the patron achieved powerful orgasm. The masseur then cut the client down before he was completely strangled.

There have been some unusual measures taken against sexual deviants in society:

In ancient Rome, bestiality was not against the law, but very much frowned upon. To discourage sex with animals, a large sales tax was imposed on the sale of beasts.

Artificial stimulators have been used almost as long as the regenerative organs themselves. Mankind has been ingenious in finding objects for sexual pleasure:

The artificial penis of ancient Greece was made of either padded leather or wood. A play dating back to the third century B.C. began with a character, Metro, asking her girlfriend Coritto for her dildo.

At one time, in the ancient Far East, cat's feet were used as dildos.

In 18th-century Japan, women were skilled in the art of using the harigata, or dildo. The dildo was made of leather, wood, buffalo horn, porcelain or tortoise shell. These ingenious pleasure seekers strung cords around their necks and through the dildos. By moving their backs and shoulders, they could make the dildo move inside their bodies while using their hands to manipulate other areas.

Russian peasant women were known to tie knots in their clothing in the area of their vulvae. In this way they could masturbate against the hard knot of cloth.

During the Edo period (17th century) in Japan, decorative masks, known as kagura, were commonly hung on the walls. These masks often featured Tenggu, a goblin with a very large nose. As well as being decorative, these masks were functional. Tenggu's nose could be removed and used as a dildo.

In ancient India, it was common for pleasure-seeking males to cut small incisions in their penises, insert little round balls, and let the incisions heal. The sensation of the little balls underneath the skin of the penis greatly enhanced the female's sexual feeling.

The Kamasutra suggested that the size of the penis could be enlarged, though temporarily. If the male could tolerate the pain, he could achieve extra size by constantly rubbing his penis with a certain insect's bristles.

Amerind girls, in an effort to increase their pleasure by thickening their partner's penis, placed poisonous bugs on the male member. The bites induced a severe swelling, for which the females were very grateful.

Borellus related an incident where a man rubbed his penis with musk before sex. This caused a reaction that prompted his wife's vagina to dilate, fiercely gripping the penis. A doctor had to be consulted to pry the two lovers apart. A large amount of water was injected to allow separation of the locked parts.

In northern Celebes, males tied goats' eyelashes to a spot just behind their glans penis. This added considerably to the stimulation of their partners.

Morga noted that women of the Pintadas Islands took special pains to ensure their satisfaction. When the boys of the tribe were young, their penises were punctured. A metal or ivory snake head, along with a wedge, was placed under the skin and left to heal. This was a great source of pleasure to the women and was known as sagra.

The East Indian used many kinds of attachments inserted into the hole punched into the penis. These erotic toys were called apadravyas and were made of many different materials: buffalo horn, copper, gold, iron, ivory, lead, tin, silver or wood. There were just as many different styles: the round, the round on one side, the wooden mortar, the flower, the armlet, the bone of the heron, the goad of the elephant, the collection of eight balls and others.

Bisayos in the Philippines pierced their penises and inserted a tiny lead bar horizontally. Attached to the ends of the bar were little star-shaped objects that spun about. Upon penetration, the woman felt a certain amount of pain, but apparently it was little enough compared to the erotic excitement the spinning stars produced.

The East African Nandi men discovered a plant called yeptiringuet which was an effective aid to masturbation. The plant juice was milky and sticky, and caused an irritation that enlarged the glans penis, pulling the foreskin back.

In the mid-16th century, a Venetian reported that the Arab girls in the harems of Constantinople were carefully watched. When served cucumbers, for instance, it was expressly forbidden to have a cucumber enter the harem unless it was sliced. Previously, the girls had used the cucumbers to satisfy themselves sexually.

Men in ancient Japan utilized a plant to enhance their sex lives. The plant had long, stringy threads. The man bound his penis in this plant. When it dried, it took the form of a penis-cast. The man had sex with his lover, and the moisture of her vagina made the cast swell and expand. The reduction of friction on the penis with this cast made the erection last longer and prolonged his pleasure. The increased size of his member pleased the woman.

The Trukese women of the Pacific found pleasure in inserting the meat of coconuts into their vaginas and having a dog eat it out.

A Chinese writer of the 14th-century Ming dynasty was T'ao Tsung-i. He reported the use of a plant for women's sexual pleasure. The plant was called So-Yang. It was similar to a pointed bamboo shoot, with a scaly texture. In many ways, it resembled the human penis. Women inserted this shoot into their vaginas. The plant, when moistened, expanded, causing a great amount of pleasure for the ancient Chinese women.

China was home to a plant called Mien-Ling. This little plant was shaped like a conical bell. Inside was a small bean or seed. Once heated, the little object inside the plant twitched and bounced, not unlike the Mexican Jumping Bean. The vibration of the Burma Bell provided great sexual excitement to the ladies who introduced the plant into their vaginas.

During the late Manchu dynasty, manufacturers created Mr. Horn. Mr. Horn was made of rubber. The erotic device was similar in concept to a hot water bottle, but very distinctly phallus-shaped. Later, Mr. Horn was combined with a belt so that one woman could play the male, while the other received Mr. Horn.

Nineteenth-century girls and women were so persistent in using (and losing) hairpins to masturbate that in 1860 an English surgeon patented a surgical instrument specially designed to remove hairpins from vaginas.

In ancient China it was common practice to stuff dried mushrooms into small bags. The expansion of the packet of dried mushrooms under the moisture and heat of the vagina was a pleasure frequently indulged in.

The ever-ingenious Chinese created sexual toys in the 12th and 13th centuries such as the double olishos, a dildo that could accommodate two women at once. The device was an ivory or wooden phallus with two silk belts in the middle of it. The movement of one woman created pleasure for the other.

Another device was a dildo that could be manipulated by moving the heel of the foot. This kept the hands free for other amorous activities, or perhaps household duties.

The Aaru Archipelago Islands were occupied by a tribe that practiced surgery on the male to increase the woman's pleasure during intercourse. The procedure was a modified circumcision whereby the upper piece of foreskin was removed. The women of the islands definitely favored those men who had the alteration.

The East African Kikuyu boys who could tolerate two painful sessions to show their courage were circumcised in two stages. The first stage involved cutting the foreskin off the tops of their penises. The bottom part of the foreskin was removed later. Between the two operations, the second half of the foreskin was left to rot. During this time, females were eager to have sex with these boys. They experienced extreme sexual pleasure as a result of this partial operation.

In Egypt the pleasures of anal sex were quite common. It is no wonder, then, that they had certain erotic experts called Shepherds of the Anus.

Sir Richard Burton noted the inclination toward bestiality that the Egyptian men practiced, at least up to the 19th century. They rolled female crocodiles on their backs so as to render them immobile. The Egyptian men then mounted the crocodiles. They believed that mating with crocodiles attracted the good fortune of the gods. It was especially recommended to older men, as the mating with female crocodiles was supposedly a cure for old age.

Adornment of the body for sexual enhancement has a long and venerable history. However, clothing has also been used by the sexually inhibited for the opposite effect:

In old Ireland, sex was the source of extreme embarrassment and guilt. To reduce the feeling of sensual pleasure and its attendant guilt, it was common practice for sexual partners to indulge in intercourse without actually removing their underwear.

The pursuit of pleasure has been well organized:

In London in 1670, a club called The Dancing Club was formed. This title told only half the story. The members of this club were men and women of loose morals. The members used the music and merriment to get their blood moving—in anticipation of later securing a room upstairs for the close contact dancing. To ready themselves, the men and women were content to "shake their rumps and exercise their members to some tune."

Men's clubs in 17th-century England did little in the way of public service. On the contrary, most clubs offered organized adventures in violence and sex. Information on brothels and whores was vigorously exchanged between members and clubs.

Each club had its own specialty. The Mohocks liked to beat people up and sexually humiliate women. The Bold Bucks spent most of their time raping women. The Sweaters occupied their time by using their swords on citizens. The Blasters explored every possibility of exposing themselves. The Fun Club played nasty tricks and practical jokes on unsuspecting passersby. The members of a club called The Mollies enjoyed dressing as women.

In Scotland in 1732, the nobility and gentry of the districts of Fife and Caledonia met in the Castle Dreel in Anstruther. Twice a year, on St. Andrew's Day and Candlemas, they convened as The Beggar's Benison.

The initiation of new members was unique. The candidate, attended to by a Recorder and two Remembrancers, closeted himself. He then masturbated himself to full erection. He was then escorted into the club's meeting room to four triumphant blasts of a horn. On an altar sat the Testing-Platter.

The greenhorn was obliged to place his penis on the platter, whereupon the size of his erection was measured and noted in a book. Then his lodge brothers approached him two by two. They exposed their erect penises, and one by one, touched erect penises with the newcomer. This ceremony was presided over by a Sovereign, who wore a wig supposedly woven from the pubic hairs of the mistresses of Charles II. The initiate then read a passage from *The Song of Solomon*, including various comments and opinions he might have on the erotic piece.

After this took place, the banquet started. These were noisy, gay affairs, with obscene toasts and lascivious songs dominating the conversation. At some point a toast was made to the new member, allowing him license to, as a ship's captain might, "navigate the narrow channels" he might come across in his travels. After the banquet, the members occupied themselves in other erotic matters. Sometimes the members "frigged" themselves, comparing the length of time to achieve orgasm and the result of the masturbation. At each meeting, the wig was passed around, kissed and worn for a short time by each member.

The club also sponsored nubile young women between 14 and 19 to enter the meeting chambers naked except for a shawl over the face. The girls laid down, spread-eagled on their backs, and then on their stomachs. In a very orderly manner, the "Knights passed in turn and surveyed the Secrets of Nature."

The club had its final meeting on St. Andrews Day, 1836.

In 18th-century France, a restricted club (membership: 200 only) called The Aphrodites practiced sexual indulgence. The membership was variable. Rabbis, monks, society men, financiers, musicians, valets, army officers, bishops, abbots and princes were just some of the many club members. Initiates paid a membership fee—the equivalent of $3,500 for men and $1,200 for women. This was a considerable sum in the 18th century, when a servant could earn as little as $50 a year.

Once each Aphrodite applicant fulfilled the monetary requirements, there was the matter of the physical requirement. The new member proved his or her eligibility by being able to make love continuously for many hours—while being observed by the "admissions committee."

Because of the club's wealth, their headquarters, a country home, was beautifully and functionally landscaped and furnished for all passionate possibilities.

One of these custom-designed furnishings was the Avantageuse. This structure supported the female in the sexual encounter. She lay back on a narrow satin "mattress" that supported her from her head to the small of her back. She grabbed columns on either side of her—the columns carved to represent two tall phalluses. Two footrests were set slightly forward of her reclining back, allowing her to recline further. These stirruplike footrests were set far apart, to spread-eagle her legs.

The man approached the reclining partner from the front. He rested his knees on a bar between her legs, which placed his genitals on level with hers. He balanced himself by placing his hands on hand rests on either side of the woman.

The members enjoyed many opportunities for lovemaking. One woman, a 20-year member, noted 4,959 sexual connections with men.

The primitive approach to organized and group-sex encounters has usually been very playful:

Trobriand Islanders of the southern part of the island mixed sport and sex. Single men lined up on one side of a rope, women on the other. They then engaged in a tug-of-war. When one team collapsed, the winners insulted them with the katugogva, or victory scream. Then they charged the losers, still on the ground, and initiated sex until an orgy began.

Tourists to ancient Mexico discovered the natives practicing an ingenious method of doubling their pleasure:

The History of the Conquest of Mexico, written by Bernal Diaz del Castillo, noted an interesting method of sexual indulgence. The ancient Mexicans were in the habit of inserting funnels into their anuses and pouring wine into their rectums. As well as sexually exciting the natives, it also made them drunk.

Among the Arabs of Oman, it was acceptable for men to have intercourse with camels, cows or sheep. However, after he had taken his pleasure, the milk produced by the animal was considered tainted. For this reason, the men were obligated to kill the animals they had sex with.

The human mind has been ingenious in the pursuit of pleasure:

As recently as 1985, in Texas, people practiced gerbillophilia. Those who practiced gerbillophilia found sexual excitement by inserting a funnel of sorts into their anuses. A live rodent, a gerbil, was put into the funnel. The gerbillophiliac waited for the gerbil to make its way into the anus, then pulled the funnel out. The little rodent struggled to make its way out of the anus. The movement of the gerbil in the rectum apparently produced great pleasure for the gerbillophiliac.

Severe judgments have been taken against those who challenged religious authority and its opposition to sensual pleasure:

In the third century A.D., the church proclaimed that a woman should have sex for one reason, and one reason only: to bear children. If she indulged in sex for any other reason, such as to please her husband or out of her own desires, she was considered to be a prostitute.

Sexual proficiency has been a great source of pride among primitive cultures:

The Swahilis in Zanzibar were one of the few peoples who preferred to indulge in intercourse with woman dominant. In this position, the woman squatted on top of the male. The old women taught 60 to 80 young women a hip-grinding movement for eight hours a day, through dancing naked, taking a full 40 days to three months of instruction to perfect the technique. Men were forbidden to witness this exercise.

To be unable to master this method, called digitisha, was shameful. The lowest insult one could cast on a Swahili woman was to accuse her that she was ignorant of the technique of digitisha. It was only after she had mastered this pleasure-increasing, hip-grinding movement that she was presented as a marriageable girl.

Erotic behavior has included practically every type of manipulation on every part of the body:

Hottentot men excited the female partner through an unusual form of foreplay: To increase the female's pleasure, they spanked their partners hard on the buttocks before intercourse.

Tamil lovers did not kiss each other during intercourse. Instead, they rubbed noses and licked each other's mouths and tongues.

A sexual technique particular to the Ponape and Trobriand Island lover was the practice of mitakuku. Mitakuku was the biting off of a lover's eyebrows and eyelashes and was a technique of foreplay as well as the moment of climax.

As a sign of extreme excitement and satisfaction, the Pacific Trukese woman stuck her finger in her partner's ear.

In most cultures, food, shelter and war have been primary preoccupations. There have been exceptions:

Between Needles, California, and Parker, Arizona, on the banks of the Colorado River, lived a tribe of Indians called the Mohaves. The tribespeople were very sexually indulgent. The Mohaves instructed their children to enjoy sex as often as possible before they became too old and regretted their lost opportunities.

Almost every kind of sexual activity possible was explored and practiced by the easygoing Mohaves. Normal and common sexual practices for the tribe included masturbation, mutual masturbation, fellatio, anal intercourse, exhibitionism, voyeurism, group sex, incest, male and female transvestism and homosexuality, bestiality and the most lurid obscenity in both speech and gesture.

Though by no means common, Amazon women sometimes took coati monkeys as sexual partners.

The Kurtachi men and women of the Pacific, if they could find no other partner immediately available, had sex with dogs.

In Japan, seaport prostitutes in the Hong Kong harbor offered the ultimate pleasure to a man. The service was expensive to the man and dangerous to the woman. The Sampan girl, working in a boat, leaned over the side of the boat and ducked her head into the water. The customer entered her from behind, experiencing exquisite vaginal spasms around his penis as the woman reacted to her near-drowning. She pulled herself out of the water just before she lost consciousness, usually after the client had experienced an intense orgasm.

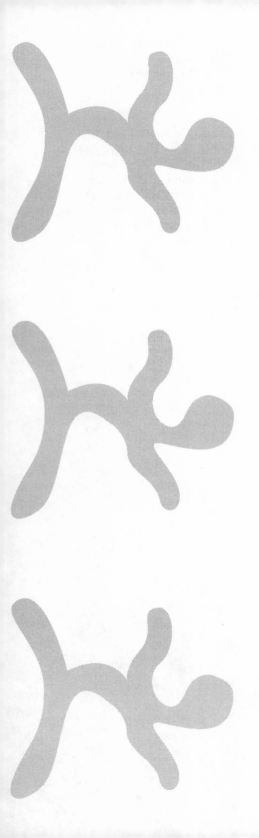

Fidelity and Adultery

St. Ambrose (A.D. 339–397), Bishop of Milan, declared that all men and women should remain virgins for the rest of their lives.

~⊙~

The South Indian Toda man was considered immoral if he refused to share his wife with other men.

~⊙~

The British Columbian Haida husband could not take vengeance on his adulterous wife or her lover. However, the lover was obligated to pay damages—not to the husband, but to his lover's mother.

~⊙~

The King's cook in Angoi was not allowed to have sexual relations while employed by the king.

~⊙~

The Bahima girls of Ankole were very carefully guarded and were practically kept under house arrest. If a girl slept with a man, the punishment was death by drowning. However, after she was married, her husband lent her out, and she took on lovers.

On the Fruit Mellori and Nicobar Islands, adultery was severely punished if it occurred between members of different classes of people. However, if the couple were of the same caste, a wife could be lent out if the husband was given a token such as a leaf of tobacco.

During the Sioux festival to bring forth the buffalo in the spring, young

Sioux men gave their wives to the old men, who had intercourse with them.

Among some tribes of Venezuela, marriage did not immediately affect a person's availability. A married man or woman could have sex with another person in the first year of their marriage. It was not until they had been married a year that they were required to be faithful.

~O~

Complete sexual freedom has been bestowed on a select few in most societies—and sometimes it is surprising who these people were:

The court jesters of the Middle Ages enjoyed almost complete sexual freedom. Thought of as less than human, as idiots and fools, their behavior, no matter how outrageous, was merely laughed at and discounted.

Thus, they could get away with every sort of flirting, obscenity, and sexual prank. Their special untouchable status, as well as their clever tongues and good humor, made them extremely popular with the ladies of the courts.

The fool's freedom of speech and behavior was often so sexually explicit that in 789 the church refused any clergyman permission to keep a jester.

~O~

Occasionally a change in mates has been not by inclination, but by obligation:

The Turkish courtier was often rewarded by his sultan with the gift of the sultan's daughter. He had to build a palace for his new bride. He got no dowry from the sultan except for a diamond-studded dagger—which she kept as a token of her superiority over him. As the sultan's daughter, she had complete control over his life. He had to get rid of all his wives and concubines, and he was not allowed to turn down the offer of the princess's hand.

~O~

Kissing was not a common expression of affection of the Burundi. When a man kissed a woman, it was assumed that he had committed adultery with her. As punishment, the man's lower lip was cut off.

~O~

At one time, priests and nuns were housed in common areas. This practice, however, was very short-lived:

In the Middle Ages, the Church briefly instituted the practice of building nunneries and monasteries together, with only a wall between the two sexes' lodgings. This revealed to the church administration a disturbing reality. In very short order, every one of the "brides of Christ" had become pregnant—even though the nuns far outnumbered the monks.

~⊙~

Clement of Alexandria (A.D. 150–215) declared that "one commits adultery with one's own wife if one has commerce with her in marriage as if she were a harlot."

~⊙~

While certain sexual behavior was frowned upon by society, moralists could not ignore the reality of the situation:

France of the 1300s took bastardy in stride. While the church was absolutely opposed to the occurrence, moralists advised that the bastard child be accepted. Typical of this attitude was the Chevalier De La Tour Landry. In an instructional book dedicated to his daughters, Landry encouraged wives to raise their husband's children by other women.

~⊙~

What some cultures might term adultery has been a natural part of the cultural makeup of another society:

The Fiji Island Melanesian kings had especially devoted wives. The king's wife did the usual tasks a mate performed. But she had another very important duty. She chose a child who showed great promise of beauty and grace from among the villagers. For the next many years, she devoted all her time and energy to raising the girl.

The adoptee was eventually to become the king's mistress. When fully mature and ready to be presented, the king's wife removed the girl's clothes, beautified her with a bath and perfume and fixed her hair. Then the king's wife led the mistress, naked, to her husband, for his pleasure.

~⊙~

A great number of the world's cultures have been polygamous, and the women of these cultures accepted this structure quite willingly:

Among the Nigerian Ibos, men had several wives. Women were more eager to be one of several wives than to be the lone wife of a man. One-woman men were considered weak of character and far less desirable.

A Zambian man had to formally get his wife's permission before taking a lover. However, a wife was obliged never to oppose her husband's wishes.

~⊙~

Having many wives while providing sexual variety had its responsibilities. Attached to the luxury of novelty was the obligation to satisfy:

In ancient China, a man had a moral obligation to satisfy all his wives and concubines sexually. In the Confucian Book of Rites, called Li-Chi, he was instructed to lay with each of his concubines at least every fifth day. This was their right, and his duty.

~O~

The man entitled to many wives often had the problem of being an attentive lover to all who shared his bed. In some cases, elaborate plans were followed to satisfy the needs of the participants:

Chinese royalty had a very orderly system to ensure the pleasure of the ruler and his women. The proper number of mates he was allowed was based on a very old system of numbers magic. His companions: one queen, three consorts, nine second-rank wives, 27 third-rank wives and 81 concubines.

In addition, he needed sexual bookkeepers, who kept a schedule of who was entitled to go to bed with the king on a particular night. The tabulators recorded the day and hour of each encounter in their erotic ledgers. This cycle was usually ascendant, starting with the lowest concubine and working up to the queen. This particular order was religiously followed.

Supposedly the queen benefited from the king's consorting with the previous 120 women, because his powers would be at their highest while with her. The benefit she received was definitely not in frequency, however. She bedded the king only once a month, at the end of the cycle of women.

The ancient Japanese shogun's sexual encounters were known as otawa-mure—"august dalliance." The performance of these dalliances was very formal. The concubine was notified that she was to sleep with the shogun. For this occasion, she always wore a pure white silk kimono.

At about 9 a.m. she was led to a room adjoining the shogun's and female attendants removed her clothes, checking for possible weapons. Her hair was taken down, with the hairpins (as possible weapons) replaced by a comb. The shogun made his appearance an hour later, receiving kneeling bows from his matrons. They then departed, with the exception of one, who stayed in an adjoining room to witness the coupling.

~O~

One of the world's greatest polygamists was King Solomon (955–935 B.C.), who supposedly had 700 wives and 300 concubines.

~O~

The East Indian woman of the Oddars could make love only to her husband. However, during her lifetime, the Oddar woman could have as many as 18 husbands.

206

In the time of Chevalier De La Tour Landry, in 13th-century France, a club of men and women called the Galois and Galoisies practiced a special version of hospitality. Whenever a fellow Galois came to the house of another Galois, the host offered the sexual services of his Galoisie, for the length of his stay.

~◉~

The King of Ashanti was allowed to have only a certain number of wives. This restriction caused few problems, however. He was restricted to having no more than 3,333.

~◉~

In the other extreme, monogamy has been vigorously enforced among cultures that held it dear:

The Tahitian girl who was promised marriage was called Vahinepahio. Since she was considered spoken for, her purity was carefully guarded. She was always waited on by a member of the family. She was never alone, except at night. Within her parents' yard was a platform, high in a tree. Here she spent most of her time of engagement, away from the threat of any claims by another man.

~◉~

Any encounters between Arapesh men and women outside the village were viewed with caution. The Arapesh considered them as seductions—opportunities for illicit lovemaking. The men were warned by their mothers against putting themselves into such a position where a woman might approach them. The belief was that men outside the village boundaries could be taken advantage of.

~◉~

Once a first-century Tapyrian husband had acquired three children by his wife, he was obliged to leave her to pair up with another man.

~◉~

The King of the Medge in the Congo punished the man who seduced one of his wives by mutilating the seducer, then killing him. However, the adulterer could save his life if he provided the king with two wives.

~◉~

Power has always meant privilege. This has especially been true in a sexual sense:

Solon (630–560 B.C.), the Athenian lawmaker, made it law that the state should have the strongest and healthiest children possible. To accomplish this, any young man who was better built than another could demand permission to sleep with the weaker man's wife.

The Trobrianders were a monogamous people. However, multiple mates were tolerated among the higher class. Sorcerers and headsmen were obligated to have several mates. Because of their special status, they were expected to have a harem of female companions.

Among the South Indian Todas, the dairy men were considered religious priests, or palol. If a man served 18 years as a palol, he was allowed to have sex in broad daylight with the woman of his choice.

Following the example of Catherine the Great (1729–1796) of Russia, who had many male lovers, it became all the rage in Russia for women of the court to hire lovers. Men became courtesans, selling their affections, in a very dignified manner, to the highest bidder.

~◉~

During the time of the Renaissance, an Italian bride could demand the right to have a lover as one of the clauses in her marriage contract.

~◉~

Among the ancient Hebrews, a married man could have an adulterous affair with an unmarried girl—provided that her father was dead.

~◉~

In the 12th century in the Middle East, women had few opportunities to entertain lovers. They had very little freedom of movement. One of the few places a woman could go was the graveyard. For this reason, this place of rest for the dead was a popular spot for some very lively sexual activities by the living.

~◉~

There have been curious blends of extreme restriction of privileges and then unexpected freedoms of the greatest kind:

Moslem wives led a very restrictive life due to all the rules imposed on their behavior. But aside from all the restrictions of being a married woman, she was given her due. Among some tribes, each year she was allowed to leave her husband for one month. The woman could go where she pleased, no questions asked.

~◉~

It is possible to find places where infidelity was carefully scheduled:

Arabs in southern Khartoum, the Assanii, had a very liberal custom regarding marital fidelity. Wives were entitled to do as they pleased for one day out of every four. They chose whomever they wished to sleep with on those days, and their choice was accepted and respected.

~⊙~

Some Brazilian tribes, when taking prisoners of war, fed their captives well and even provided them with temporary wives for sexual comfort. Then they ate the prisoners.

~⊙~

The Zaparos lover of Ecuador who stole a woman away from her husband hid out with her. Should they be seen around the village after running away, the angry husband vented his fury on the couple. They laid low, and within a short period of time the husband took another wife. Then the couple returned, and there were no hard feelings.

The Bangala of the upper Congo had a simple solution for adultery. Should a man and woman commit adultery and refuse to stop, the two men were obligated to switch wives. The innocent husband and wife of the adulterers had no say in the matter.

In Guinea, the Apingi man who committed adultery and was caught by his lover's husband spent the rest of his life as the man's slave. If his wife was caught with another woman, the lover became the husband's mistress.

~⊙~

Many cultures have recognized the right of families to share sexual favors, even while being morally strict under any other circumstances:

In Iceland in 1707, the population was drastically reduced by a terrible epidemic. To counteract the loss of life, the King of Denmark declared it an act of the greatest patriotism if women produced illegitimate children. Each woman was allowed to have six illegitimate children. A few years later the king had to forbid illegitimate births; the women had worked so well that Iceland faced overpopulation.

~⊙~

The majority of the world's cultures have allowed relations between brothers- and sisters-in-law:

Tribes living on the Tully and Pennefeather Rivers in Australia practiced sexual polygamy. When a man married a woman, he was allowed sexual access to all her sisters—whether they were married or not.

The African Banyankole and Bakitara tribes had liberal views toward marital fidelity. A husband freely shared his wife's sexual abilities with his tribal brothers.

North of Manchuria lived the Gilyak people. When a man left his wife for any length of time, on a journey or for whatever reason, his younger brother was allowed to enjoy his wife sexually. However, should the younger brother leave his wife, the elder brother was not allowed sexual access to his sister-in-law.

~⊙~

Sharing females has been a very common feature of the world's sexual practices. Many times it was not kinship, but pure hospitality, which inclined husbands to lend out their women:

A Yemen tribe, the Merekedes, practiced wife sharing. The man who had an overnight guest offered his wife for the guest's comfort and pleasure.

This politeness was offered to him regardless of the woman's looks or age. If the guest was appreciative of the woman, he was well treated. If not, the ungrateful guest was hurried away, with the bottom part of his cloak cut off.

~⊙~

Among the Tupi of Brazil and the Tocantin of the Maranhao, there was little jealousy of wandering wives. However, fathers were very jealous of their daughters' sexual exploits.

~⊙~

The practice of exchanging bedmates could also take the form of a club activity:

Herero men in South Africa shared wives. Men formed groups of mate-sharing couples. The male could not join the group unless he had a woman to trade, and brothers, perhaps because of the incest taboo, were not allowed to join the same "club."

The Bohindu man of the Congo was not allowed to have sex with his new wife until after she had become pregnant. In the meantime, she slept with whoever she pleased to get herself pregnant.

~⊙~

Fortunately for some lawbreakers, persistence could overturn the societal law:

Among the Cayapans of Ecuador, incest was prohibited. The couple was shunned and the tribe's displeasure loudly proclaimed. However, should the incestuous couple prove their stubbornness in putting up with the tribal disapproval, after a period of time, the couple was considered as equal in status to other couples.

The Circassions, who lived near the Black Sea, looked very unfavorably on adultery. Adultery was punished not by law, but by custom. The husband returned the shamed woman to her parents. The parents sold her as a slave.

The Yucatan Mayans of Mexico tolerated adultery if it was casual. However, if a couple were too consistently meeting for adulterous sex, they were killed.

~⊙~

In some cultures, polygamy has been for recreation. In others, it was a physical necessity:

The Taoists suggested that sexual variety was perfectly appropriate for the Chinese man seeking physical well-being: "The more women with whom a man has intercourse, the greater will be the benefit he derives from the act. If in one night he can have intercourse with more than 10 women it is best."

~⊙~

Some girls had what might be considered the best of both worlds:

Among some Australian tribes, a girl was engaged to a boy while a baby or as a small child. The girl was, nevertheless, allowed to make love with whomever, and however often, she wished. It was only when she was married to her intended that she was obligated to be faithful. If she strayed from her husband, she was killed.

The Arapaho Indians guarded against lovers' quarrels in a unique way. A husband was forbidden to enter his own hut while his wife had male company.

~⊙~

Others jealously guarded the sexual favors of their mates. Even very simple societies had their methods of keeping married mates honest:

The Samoan men of the Southwest Pacific had a method of keeping their wives faithful which was very straightforward. In order that they may spot a cheating wife, they "branded" them. Before leaving their wives, the Samoans painted their wives on the forehead, armpits, and abdomen, with yellow "paint."

~⊙~

The bonds of marriage have often provided partners with exclusive sexual rights over each other. At other times, institutionalized adultery could be found:

In Tanzania, the Turu natives married. However, there was a formalized method of cheating on a spouse, widespread and well accepted. This was called Mbuya, or "romantic love."

The Mbuya was undertaken to provide married people with the excitement of a new and somewhat forbidden love. The lovers always met in secret, even if the whole community knew and acknowledged the lovers' relationship.

The thrill of meeting on the sly kept the romance new and exciting, unlike the circumstances of marriage. It also allowed the other spouses the dignity of not having to deal publicly with the lovers' affair.

No matter how obvious the relationship was, the husband of the cheating wife could offer no objection unless he surprised the couple in the act of sexual intercourse. Should the couple have been discovered, the woman's lover paid the offended husband 10 goats. If the relationship was incestuous, the penalty was two heifers.

~◉~

In Nicaragua a husband who had found out that his wife was cheating on him was forced to divorce her. If he didn't, he was considered to have broken the law and was punished.

In the 17th century, after attacking the French at Rhe, the English, in stripping the dead Frenchmen, discovered an interesting custom. Many of the men had ribbons tied around their penises—found out later to be good-luck charms from their mistresses.

~◉~

Adultery was often legislated against, but penalty could be avoided. Such was the case of some of the East Indians of ancient times:

The Kamasutra, the great Indian love tome, forbade seducing a married woman. This was true, unless, of course, the man was suffering such agony that it was the only way to save himself from death. The progressive stages of his love-obsession were: "love of the eye, attachment of the mind, constant reflection; sleeplessness, loss of weight, rejection of accustomed pleasures, shamelessness, madness, fainting, and, finally, death."

~◉~

In Wales in the Middle Ages, an amobyr, or dowry, was paid by a groom to his bride's king. However, if a girl was found to have lost her virginity due to a premarital fling, she was obligated to pay the dowry to the king herself.

In the 11th century in parts of Europe, a husband who caught his wife, concubine, or even mistress having sex with someone else took punishment into his own hands. The standard penalty was banishment of the woman to a leper colony.

Adultery could be forgiven in some cases:

Many of the Moslem women caught in the act of adultery could talk their way out of the humiliation. Folklore told of possession by the magical Jinn. These amorous spirits, who possessed her while she was in passion, were irresistible, so the woman was forgiven her sin.

Because it was common for the Moslem to believe in spirit-lovers, it was a compliment to hear: "May God copulate with thee! May a thousand huge-membered virile Jinn [spirits] have carnal knowledge of thee!"

Belief in the amorous ghosts of sleep had a very real effect on those who had dream-lovers. Some Moslems believed in their dream-lovers as absolutely real. Many men and women became jealous if their lovers were suspected of carrying on an affair with a Jinn dream-lover. Some men and women apparently even delayed marriage to a real lover because they preferred the passions of their dream-lovers.

Women were the initiators of adulterous affairs among the Ecuadoran Cayapans. The punishment for adultery was whipping. Very often, however, a single girl who had an adulterous affair with a married man was spared punishment. Instead, her actions were believed to have been the result of a desire to be married. Instead of whipping the adultress, the tribe merely found her a husband.

St. Basil, a priest in the late fourth century A.D., established the church's position on the matter of adultery. If a married man had sex with a married woman, it was considered adultery, and the offended wife was obligated to refuse her husband back. If a married man had sex with an unmarried woman, it was only fornication, and the wife was obligated to take him back.

The incest taboo has helped regulate adulterous behavior:

Among the East Indian Chitrals, a man suspected of adultery was obliged to follow a ritual that cured him of his desire for the woman he had maintained an affair with.

This ritual made the woman the lover's foster mother and thus off limits to him. This ritual was simple but always worked: The man was forced to put his lips to the woman's breast.

The more aggressive approaches to adultery were less forgiving:

The northern Japanese Ainu punished adultery by levying fines and flogging. On occasion an adulterous male was hung up by his hair, with the tips of his toes just touching the ground.

The Crow Indian husband of the western plains could punish his unfaithful wife by slashing her face with his knife, or letting his tribal brothers have sex with her.

In Colonial America, the Puritan adulterers were obliged to confess their sin and beg forgiveness in front of the church congregation. They also had to pay fines or endure whippings. A more severe penalty was to have the letters AD burned onto the forehead.

When a couple were discovered to have committed adultery in ancient India, the punishment was severe. Usually the woman was subjected to harsher treatment. She was commonly publicly flogged or stoned to death. The man, for his part, had to endure the pain of a pepper-stalk jammed up his anus.

Often, the Indian male was spared death only to face it later. For those not satisfied with the justice handed out to the adulterer, there was Ilahee-intigaum, or Divine Vengeance. If this occurred, the adulterer could look forward to being abducted, castrated, and tied to a jackass. He was paraded in the streets until the effects of castration bled him to death. His body was then taken to the dung heaps and tossed in to rot with the corpse of his mistress.

Punishment of adulterers included a variation of "An eye for an eye, a tooth for a tooth":

West African Dahomians punished adultery by allowing the men and women who were cheated on to indulge in sex with each other.

The standard way to punish an unfaithful Crow Indian wife was to have her husband choose a fellow tribesman. The unfaithful wife was obligated to have sex with the husband's choice. The husband's choice, of course, was usually the ugliest and most dim-witted man of the tribe.

The women of the Marianne Islands displayed an uncommon unity in dealing with philandering husbands. The women banded around the offended wife in a most loyal and vicious manner. The husband who cheated on his wife was attacked by all the women of the tribe. They destroyed his belongings and killed him.

Ancient Roman women who were found to be adulterous were obliged as punishment to satisfy any and all men who approached them sexually. A lottery was held to decide who would be the first to lay with them.

~**O**~

Countercultures have typically used sex as a tool of rebellion—usually in advocating free love. However, it is extremely rare for a societal institution to be allowed to advocate deviancy:

An institution in Tahiti and the Society Islands, consisting of the social elite, existed as a kind of religious "lodge." The disciples of the religion, the Arioi, preached against marriage and in favor of uninhibited intercourse.

This traveling troupe of sensualists performed obscene theatrical acts and invited the onlookers to participate in the lusty free-for-all that followed. Each member took an iron-clad oath to kill any offspring of these activities and vowed never to marry. As well, no member of the group could refuse another's advances.

~**O**~

Sexual conduct has been regulated by the threat of loss of fertility, whether it be on the part of the couple engaging in sex, or the crops they relied on as food:

The Mundugumor of New Guinea had a belief that was created to regulate illicit sexual conduct within the village. This belief would thus minimize nonmarital intercourse.

The Mundugumors believed that should lovers have intercourse in any of the village's gardens, the yams in those gardens, displeased, would "leave" the garden. Instead of restricting adulterous behavior, however, it seems to have merely enhanced the thrill of this forbidden sex.

~**O**~

Superstition and simple medical ignorance have been the cause of much of the world's marital troubles:

If a Mandingo woman's breast milk ran out while she was nursing a child, she was accused of infidelity to her husband and could be divorced.

~**O**~

In most cultures, the offspring of forbidden intercourse was a natural target for disapproval. However, in other cultures, this was not so:

The Renaissance French admired the bastard child rather than condemned him. The child born a bastard was regarded as special.

Brantome expressed the French sentiment of the time this way: "These improvised children produced by stealth are far more gallant than those produced heavily, dully, and at leisure."

Bouchet agreed, saying that these children were wittier and braver because the immediate and passionate lovemaking made them "more conducive to wit and courage."

The clergy also found their pleasure on the road:

A certain kind of holy men in medieval England, called The Wandering Friars or Limitours, were notorious for their sexual escapades with wives and daughters of the villages and towns they passed through.

A certain Huguenot published an attack on the holy men of France in 1581. The name of the document was *Le Traite de Polygamie Sacree*, and it included some damning statistics. The Huguenot was indignant over the extent to which the ecclesiastics were enjoying fleshly pursuits supposedly forbidden them. In his survey of Lyons, France, the Huguenot identified 65,230 men of the cloth. He numbered their sexual partners at 67,888, and bastard children from their dalliances at 59,138. He also counted 2,083 holy men as sodomites.

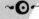

Periodic promiscuity, common among primates, has also been practiced by human beings:

The North African Barbary Macques practiced prolonged sexual activity. While the women had their periods, it was common for them to have intercourse as often as four times an hour. This continued for several days on end, by which time the women had coupled with every male in the tribe.

Rape has been almost universally taboo. However, in at least one culture, rape was essentially unknown:

With the exception of gang rape, used to punish an offending female, the New Mexican Mohaves did not have such a behavior. Because the women were so ardent for intercourse at all times, and the society so sexually oriented, rape by a single partner was unknown.

In addition, because of the sexual freedom of the tribe's women, the Mohaves did not have any form of prostitution. It was only when the white men came that the Mohave women ever sold their bodies.

THE CHASTITY PROTECTORS

One of the most well known but mysterious sexual practices has been the use of the chastity belt to ensure fidelity. The earliest known method of protecting the chastity of a woman, whether with her consent or against her will, has been infibulation:

The practice of sewing the labia majora together to prevent sexual penetration originates in Africa, with citizens of the East and Far East being early practitioners of this method.

Among many African tribes, the female was assured of keeping her virginity to marriage through means of an operation. As a young girl, her legs were spread, and the labia were scraped raw. A small reed was inserted into the vagina to allow urine to pass. The raw, bleeding labia were pressed together, and the girl's thigh's bound tightly together, so that the labia would grow together. Before she was married, a matron took a knife and cut the labia apart.

Sexual jealousy has provoked outrageous measures to protect against infidelity:

To prevent tampering with wives, the Sudanese harems were carefully protected. Once having been bedded by the master, bells were attached to the girl's wrists and ankles. A foot-long stick of bamboo was strapped to the girl's waist and thighs, and four inches of the rod thrust into her vagina. Across the vulva was placed a thatched straw mat. The bamboo pole made it difficult for her to walk. The quiet tinkling of bells assured the master that she was not indulging in a vigorous bout of sex.

A more humane method of protecting the hymen was the wearing of the "virginal belt":

In the time of Christ, copper or gold chastity belts called koomz were worn by women. Written evidence of these belts is found in the ancient Beth Haredem Nidd, 8:9: "The history of the girdle of chastity is the history of locking up the vital portal that leads to the home of virtue."

It is assumed that the belt was used to keep the woman from offering herself to another:

The word *koomz*, according to Rabbi Shelomo Izaki (born A.D. 1040), is derived from the letters of three words: *kahn*, *mokolm* and *zimo*. The three words meant "place of illicit intercourse."

There has been some argument as to whether the belts protected the woman from unwanted advances, or protected the sexual rights of the man who secured the belt. Apparently, the Greeks used theirs to protect women from unwanted advances:

The ancient Greeks employed a chastity belt made of wool, supposedly from a virgin sheep. The sash was secured with a knot called the Hurculean Knot. The knot was loosened on the wedding night. Apparently these sashes were worn not to prevent the women from satisfying themselves, but to protect them. It is believed that for the most part, the girls wore them willingly.

The Spanish men, on the other hand, were believed to have used the belt in spite of their women's wishes:

The Spanish gypsy women wore something like a handkerchief arranged about their hips and pudenda. In a culture that highly prized female sexual innocence, or *lacha ye trupos*, it protected the girls from their own desires. It was regularly checked to ensure that it had not been tampered with.

⚜

The extent to which chastity belts were worn is not well known; only the metal belts have survived the years, and there is reason to believe that many specimens were destroyed or buried with the bearer who had died:

Aside from the belts made in the 1800s, there are only a few hundred chastity belts in existence. Of these, there are a number dating from the 1500s and 1600s. But only two chastity belts have survived that date back before the Renaissance.

In 1889, the corpse of a woman dating from the 1600s was found in the vault of an old church. Under her funeral dress was attached a chastity belt.

The references to the practice of wearing chastity belts, both in literature and in court records, indicated that the belts were worn more for the male's peace of mind than to protect a woman from an undesirable advance.

The earliest literary record of the chastity belt as it appeared in the time after the Crusades is in a 1405 work called *Bellifortis*.

The chastity belt was responsible for the birth of the word *trousers*:

Saint Amant testified that Roman women of the 1600s wore "a trowse of iron," thus creating the word *trowsers*, which was later incarnated into the word *trousers*.

The chastity belt may be considered a breakthrough in the fashion sense:

The chastity belt was the first form of underwear worn by Christians—specifically women.

The metal chastity belt was a simple idea with many variations:

The most basic design of the Girdle of Chastity was a two-part contraption. It merely consisted of a band of flexible metal and perforated pair of hinged plates.

The more elaborate, comfortable models were usually built thusly:

> The grille of gold hangs from four little steel chains, encased in rough silken cloth, which are joined in the same way to a belt of similar metal.
>
> The grille is supported both in front and behind by these four chains, two on one side and likewise two on the other. Above the loins the belt is linked together by a fastener for which a very small key is adapted.
>
> The grille is about six inches high and three inches broad, thus extending from the perineum to the upper margin of the external lips...and covers the whole of that region which extends from between the thighs to the lower part of the belly. As the grille is fitted with three bars it permits the passage of urine but prevents access even to the tips of the fingers.

Some chastity belts were made of leather rather than hinged metal:

Colonial Pennsylvanian women were subjected to chastity belts. The heavy leather belt was studded with rivets, and the posterior hooked on to the pubic shield by a padlock. These were called either Einholder, "restrainer" or Futsashdupper, "private organ shield."

Cireassian girls from the age of 10 were fitted with a kind of chastity belt. It was a kind of corset, or, in some cases, a more sturdy girdle made of untanned leather. The poorer girls had the belt sewn into place around their bodies. The wealthier girls were protected by tiny silver locks. The belt was removed only on the girl's wedding night. The groom carried a knife to bed to release his new wife. Considering the groom's eagerness and excitement, for the bride this could often be a risky operation.

The modern metal version of the belt was based on the devices used in the ancient Far East:

The chastity belt is believed to have been introduced to Europe by the soldiers returning from the Crusades in the 11th to 13th centuries. The medieval warriors brought back many erotic devices and ideas following this war, which was fought to curb the spread of paganism and to prove the rightness of the Christian way of life. Ironically, the Christians instead adopted many of the East's "heathen" ideas and attitudes.

A single man is believed to be responsible for the spread of the popularity of chastity belts in Europe:

The first individual associated with the European metal chastity belt was a tyrant from Venice, Italy: Francesco II, Novello Carrara. Executed in 1406 for political reasons after a lifetime of assorted cruelties, Carrara was the first man known to have kept his mistress in the Girdle.

There was some confusion over the belt's European origins:

A certain Lacroix held the idea that France introduced the belt directly from the Far East after the Crusades. Others claimed that it passed through Italy, then into France by the Italians. Diderot (1713–1784) called the girdle of chastity "the Florentine [Italy] Tool."

Rabelais: "The deuce [devil], he that has no white in his eye, take me then with him, if I don't buckle my wife in the Bergemask [Turkish] fashion, when I go out for my seraglio [harem]."

The morality and effectiveness of these belts were represented in art and literature, and even on the belts themselves through engraving:

An early reference to the Girdle of Chastity was in the woodcut called *Ship of Fools*, dated 1572. It compared the man who tried to keep his wife honest by keeping her in the belt with all the other fools and idiots of the world. The woodcut represented "the fool who protects the locusts from the sun; the fool who pours water into a well; and the fool who tries to protect by force the virtue of his wife."

Aeneas Sylvius, Pope Dius II (1405–1464), remarked on the practice:

"Those jealous Italians do very ill to lock up their wives; for women are of such a disposition they will mostly covet that which is denied the most, and offered least when they have free liberty to trespass."

The belt has been used to refuse sexual titillation of any kind, from either a lover or the belt's wearer:

A German book dated 1781 noted the use of the chastity belt long before that time. Called Mudler's Girdle, it assured parents that their daughter wasn't masturbating. Apparently, female masturbation was very common.

The restrainer was a thin metal band covered with leather or padded with material. It fit snugly but was flexible and light. An arc passed between the legs and was fastened in front. A small lock secured the hinge around the girl's abdomen. They were later abandoned in favor of restrictive clothing with narrow openings.

In a work called *Prospectus*, dated 1885, a Dr. E. Dingwall suggested that the French originally used chastity belts to prevent masturbation, and only later were they introduced to protect against illicit sexual intercourse.

Men were not immune to the wearing of chastity belts:

In the early 1800s, a Frenchman, Monsieur Jalads-Lafond, was known to have been making chastity belts for over 20 years.

They consisted of a wide belt or corset made of strong woven material. To this was attached a metal box or container (to hold the genitals), of which the outer tube was perforated at the end, the sides being drilled for the purposes of ventilation. The whole thing was secured around the body by means of locks.

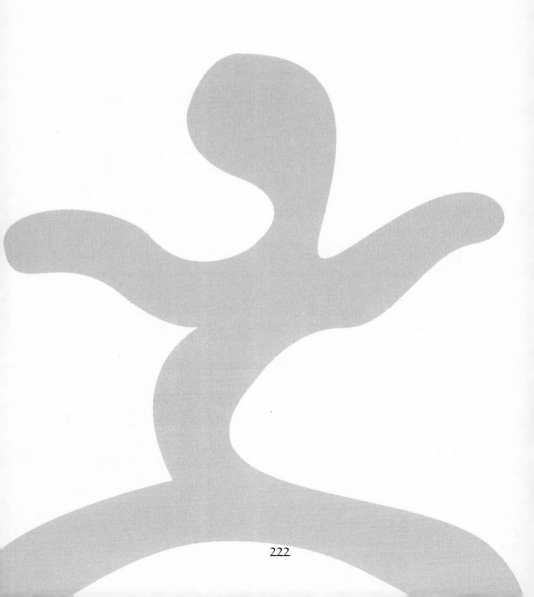

HOMOSEXUALITY AND TRANSVESTISM

The reasons for homosexual inclination have been studied and argued for thousands of years, with propositions of every sort put forth:

After studying sexual attitudes for over 30 years during the 1800s, Sir Richard Burton came to his own conclusions about homosexuality. He believed that the homosexual impulse was a matter of geographic position. This impulse was restricted to those living in areas of the world around the equator. Homosexuality was common and acceptable to people, he hypothesized, living near the equator. Burton named the area the Sotadic Zone.

Symonds thought the south of Italy to be populated with people genetically homosexual. He offered that "all the soldiers in the Italian Army have to sleep with their drawers on, even in the hottest weather, because of the indecent attacks which the Sicilians and Neapolitans habitually make on them."

Homosexual love was common among priests who had no access to women:

Sodomy among priests was such a subject of concern in 12th-century England that the church council had to issue a severe warning. It specifically threatened disciplinary action to priests who indulged in the act.

Homosexuality appears to have been around as long as heterosexuality. At many times in history, it has been perfectly acceptable:

In the sixth century B.C., in Sumeria, homosexuality was well accepted. In a book concerning astrology and sex, the region and time of Libra was for the love of a man for a woman. Pisces was the best region for the love of a woman for a man. Scorpio was the best for the love of a man for a man.

In ancient Rome, the citizenry celebrated a holiday in honor of its courtesans—every April 24, by the Roman calendar. The following day, April 25, was Fasti Praenestini, which celebrated the male prostitutes of Rome.

During the T'ang dynasty in China, it was commonplace for actors to be homosexual. In fact, while the student of drama studied his craft, he prepared himself for the eventuality of anal intercourse.

The benches that accommodated the pupils had wooden pegs sticking out of them. As the drama student progressed in his education, he grew accustomed to successively larger pegs penetrating his anus as he made his way down the bench.

Homosexual love between man and boy in ancient Greece was accepted practice. Between the teacher and the student, the Greeks believed, there had to be a bond that committed both parties to each other completely.

The eligible young boy behaved like his sister. His eyes were lowered as he walked in public. He was seen in public only with a chaperone. He avoided the less refined places: shops, the baths, the houses of Heterai or Greek courtesans. He stayed away from the common sorts of idlers, rough men and merchants. He wore a robe that looked very much like one worn by the Greek woman.

A certain kind of pottery was reserved for homosexual attachments in ancient Greece. These pieces, called Kalos vases, were given to the boys by their male lovers. The Kalos vase was never given by a man to a woman.

Often a man in love with a boy showed his devotion by having a statue of Eros erected at the boy's gymnasium or bath house.

Homosexuality has been used to great advantage by some countries:

The ancient Greeks thought that the loyalty of a man to his lover would inspire great courage. They had a group of warriors that consisted of 150 pairs of homosexual lovers. The Sacred Battalion of Thebes, as it was called, lasted 33 years and fought with distinction. It was finally wiped out at the Battle of Chaeronea by the Macedonians in 338 B.C.

Some of the most masculine of men have indulged in homosexual relations:

In Japan, from the 13th to the 19th centuries in particular, the fierce Samurai knights kept youths called kosho. The kosho were pages who submitted to the sexual embraces of their masters. This sodomy was considered a more manly release of sexual energy than with a delicate and fragile female. The pages, as a service to the Samurai knights, also sexually satisfied their master's wives.

The ancient Cretians paired veteran warriors with youths. This arrangement was called paiderastia. Before being taught the ways of war by the older warrior, the young man was taken on a romantic "honeymoon" for a few weeks.

In medieval Islam, men were given this advice concerning homosexuals: "Don't sit with the sons of the rich, for they have features like women, and they are a worse temptation than virgins."

Bisexuality has been accepted for centuries. Ancients reasoned that the opposite sex satisfied one need, the same sex, another: The ancient Islamic author Kai Ka'us ibn Iskandar wrote *Qabus-nama* in 1082. In it he suggested that the male should not choose between men and women. Instead, he recommended spending the summers with boys and the winters with women.

In ancient Persia, houses of female prostitution were nearly nonexistent. However, brothels of male prostitutes were extremely common.

Some societies practiced what amounted to periodic homosexuality:

During the Cayapan festivals, men engaged in homosexual behavior. On these occasions there was much heavy and continuous drinking. It was at these times that young men and boys would hold each other in their arms or hold hands in a very affectionate manner. After the festivals, however, life went on as usual.

Forced homosexual activity has been used as a cruel sign of contempt for, and domination over, a beaten enemy:

The Russians fought the Turks in two wars, the Crimean and the Russo-Turkish wars. The Russians were shocked by the battlefield habits of the Bashi-Bazouk, the Turkish "military bastards." These Bashi-Bazouk had a habit of dropping their pants and taking advantage of the dying enemy's anal spasms to satisfy their sexual desires.

Sodomy was a relatively commonly accepted practice among Turks:

Turkey had a particular group of men who made their living by sodomy, called the Lewwautee. Their motto was:

The penis smooth and round,
was made with the anus to match it;
Had it been for the vulva's sake,
it had been formed like a hatchet!

It has been reported that in some places, homosexuality was more common that heterosexuality:

In the part of Peru called Chimu, on the northern coast, sodomy was more popular with men than any other sexual activity. So notoriously inverted were these people that, after the Incas executed all the sodomites, the women outnumbered the men by 15 to 1.

In some cultures, female homosexuality was viewed as an inevitability, and in some cases, these relations were encouraged:

The nature of woman, along with her limited usefulness in the eyes of her husband, made female homosexuality quite acceptable in ancient China. In fact, the selfless love of one woman for another was often considered as touching as the male/female romance.

Fear of homosexuality has inspired vicious attacks against its practitioners; however, other, more intellectual arguments have been made against homosexuality:

The supposed threat of "increasingly" homosexual practices in England and Ireland in the 1700s created much concern. Homosexual behavior was so common, it was believed that it threatened the stability of the two countries. One of the appeals to return to more conventional sexual practice was called "An Essay upon Improving and Adding to the Strength of Great Britain and Ireland by Fornication."

In other places, homosexuality has been considered useful and even, at times, necessary:

The central Australian Aranda tribe had a premarriage custom that might have been useful in controlling the birth rate. Between the time a boy was initiated into manhood and the time he was married, he kept a boy. The boy was a substitute wife for the single young man. These boy-wives were usually between 10 and 12 years old.

Among some cultures, homosexuality was a rite of passage:

The Keraki tribe of Southwest New Guinea initiated their pubescent boys by making them homosexual partners to older boys. This apprenticeship started with the new initiates being passive partners. At the end of one or two years, the roles were switched between the older and younger boys. Until the boys were married, they practiced homosexual love with younger, newly initiated boys.

Homosexual practices have, in some instances, been considered indispensable for a boy's health and happiness:

Polynesian fathers asked close male relatives to help in their son's physical growth. The relative was the provider of semen to the boy, who fellated the elder to obtain all the benefits of his elder's semen.

The boys of the Ngonde tribe were segregated from the rest of the tribe. They had their own village. Homosexuality was accepted from the time the boys entered the camp, at the age of 10, until they married. Once the young men married, however, homosexuality was frowned upon, merely because by then it was viewed as a sign of immaturity.

Lebanese men were allowed to have sexual relations with female animals without penalty. But if the Lebanese male had sex with a male animal, he was put to death.

In some parts of ancient Greece, national erotic festivals occurred. Two locations particularly well known for these lusty festivals were Cithaeron and Parnassus. Women and girls dressed in costumes and climbed to a mountaintop. There they made music, drank wine and danced. Sacrifices were made, and the blood, along with the music and the alcohol (which was very potent to these nondrinkers), usually led these women to indulge in lesbian orgies.

Other cultures were less tolerant of homosexuality:

In ancient Islam, on the day of resurrection, said Ibn Abbas, the homosexual would "come out in disgrace above the heads of the crowd with his penis hung on the anus of his companion."

In 16th-century France, there were two trials involving lesbian relationships. In both cases only the woman who played the male role was punished. While the passive partner was set free, the "transvestite" was put to death.

Among the ancient Aztecs, sexual activity between lesbians and between transvestites was forbidden. Those caught engaging in this activity were punished harshly. The partners taking the active role in these sexual games were tied to a log and smothered with hot coals until death came. The partners playing the passive role suffered the same fate, as well as having their stomachs pulled out through their anuses.

During the reign of ancient Roman emperor Caligula, prostitutes wore male togas to distinguish them from the "honest" women.

Among the peasant populations in northern Albania, Montenegro and other parts of the western Balkans, transvestism was allowed. Some unmarried virgin girls assumed male dress and took manly jobs. Many of these girls assumed the male role because they were only children in the family, and it was desirable to have a male child. In some cases, the eldest daughter in a family of girls took on the role of a boy so that the younger sisters could have a brother to "protect" them.

These girls were perfectly masculine in appearance as well as behavior, many of them smoking and drinking with the other men of the village. They even joined in on commenting on the charms of attractive young village girls.

There have been some famous cross-dressers in history. Many were women trying to gain the benefits of masculinity in a male-dominant society:

Hildegunde was a young girl wandering Europe with her father, a merchant of Neuss am Rhein. Her father was killed; Hildegunde, mistaken for a boy, was given a job as a cleric in Cologne, Italy, and called herself Joseph. She returned to her native Germany. In Schonau, she settled in a monastery. It was only after a very long life as a monk, on her death in 1188, that it was learned she was actually a woman.

Joan of Arc (1412–1431) achieved sainthood partly through her transvestism. One of the charges brought against her was that she wore men's clothes. Joan's clothes and weapons were all tailor-made for her at her request. When charged with cross-dressing in Rouen in 1431, she gave up the practice. A short time later she returned to wearing male clothing, refusing to give it up, and was burned at the stake on May 30, 1431, as a lapsed heretic.

☿

During the First World War, prisoners in officer's camps passed the time by setting up theaters. Young men played female roles, and soon they were entertaining admiring male fans in the same way an actress would. They were courted by other officers and allowed privileges denied others. They were given all kinds of feminine presents: perfume, candy, jewelry and the like.

☿

Homosexual transvestites have been common enough in history to have spawned many organizations devoted to the lifestyle:

In the late 18th century in London, there existed a club devoted to such interests. Besides accommodation for sexual activities, this pederast's clubhouse, located on Clement's Lane, had other facilities.

Upon being raided by the police, it was discovered that some members of this men's club were nursing babies in bed. These babies were actually rag dolls being breastfed by gentlemen.

So accomplished at playing the part of a woman was one man that an officer from the vice squad let him go, believing him to be an innocent woman.

☿

In central Africa, in the eastern Sudan, lived a tribe called the Azande. Men between the ages of 25 and 35 were formed into groups, or vura. These men were warriors in wartime and laborers for the chief in times of peace. While the men were in these groups, they were not allowed to have women. Their Aparanga had no lovers or wives in it; they used boys as substitutes. These boys played the role of the woman in every function, including the bedchamber.

Normally unacceptable behavior may oftentimes have been forgiven on special occasions:

In fourth-century Cappadocia, men dressed "in long robes, girdles, slippers and enormous wigs" on New Year's Day. This cross-dressing drew the anger of St. Asterius.

In some instances, transsexualism has even been respected:

There were three types of people designated among the Indonesian Makassars: men, women and the kawe kawe, or "it" people.

The female kawe kawe were different from their sisters only in that they did men's work while with other females. The male kawe kawe were different. They behaved like a woman among women, but sometimes assumed the male role among other men.

On the American plains, among the Illinois and Dakota Indians, certain men wore women's clothes and, because of their different lifestyle and outlook on life, earned the respect of their fellow tribesmen. The chiefs frequently asked their advice because of their unique view of the world.

The ancient Scythians, who lived north of the Black Sea, had enarees, or anarieis: these men did women's work, acted like women and were impotent. Instead of being ridiculed and abused, they were honored by the other Scythian males. The more masculine men respected these enarees, afraid that the gods would curse them in the same way.

In parts of Pakistan and India lived a group of boys called hijra. They wore female dress and acted like girls. The hijra were skilled singers and dancers, castrated at a young age—sometimes as infants. From a young age these boys enlarged their rectums by introducing greased metal or wooden cones, which became progressively larger. Their sexual function was as passive partners in sodomy.

Among the North American Koniaga Indians of Kadiak Island, a mother often chose her finest-looking son and raised him as a female. He wore female clothing, did only domestic chores and associated with only girls and women. Between the ages of 10 and 15, the boy was married off to a wealthy tribesman.

Some men of the Bathonga tribe of Mozambique were dedicated homosexuals. When transported to Johannesburg, South Africa, to work in the mines, they were settled in all-male camps. While there were female prostitutes readily available, the Bathongas preferred males playing the part of the woman.

Out of every new group of workers entering the camp, a few boys were chosen to act as women. These boys were called tinkhentshana and spent little of their time as miners. The duties arranged for them were more domestic. These boys wore breasts carved out of wood. It was common for the Tinkhentshana to marry one of the miners.

Because of the suppression of unacceptably nonreproductive sexual lifestyles, homosexuals have had to lead their lives secretly:

In the late 18th century, London's Vere Street featured an inn named The White Swan. This was a haven for pederasts, furnished for the purpose of providing private refuge for men of this special desire.

A special set of rooms was set aside for these men. One contained four beds for couples and their particular brand of sex. Another room was furnished for all the fantasies of these men, with all the frills and toilettes of a lady. Another room was a replica of a chapel, where men "married" each other in complete style, with all the customs of the ceremony being observed.

In Japan from the 15th to the 17th centuries, young boys who played the roles of women took to the stage. These female impersonators were called onnagata ("female forms"). After their performances, they sexually offered themselves to interested audience members. Many warriors fought each other to bed a young man of this type.

These young men wore women's clothing offstage as well as on. In fact, they set the fashions for female clothing and were widely imitated by women and girls.

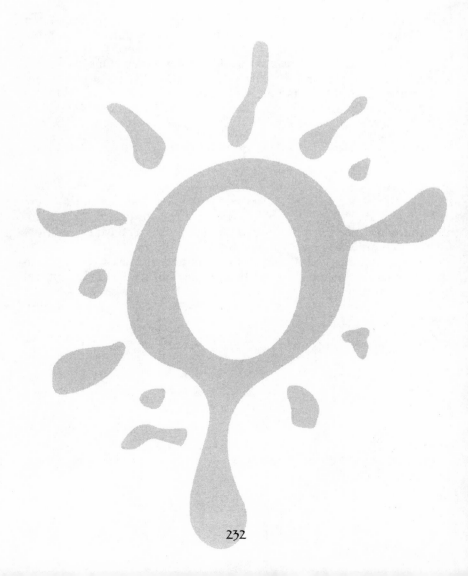

SEX AND MONEY

Chinese courtesans of the T'ang dynasty were highly thought of, and they were not treated with any less respect for making a profession out of selling their affections. In part, this was because the highly sought-after courtesan was not only attractive, but talented as well. Beauty was considered only secondary to their talents of writing, music and dance. The girl who could offer only a pretty face and a good figure was far less desirable than any of these other mannered, talented entertainers.

During World War I, some soldiers who had picked up a case of gonorrhea sold some of the resulting pus of the disease to fellow soldiers. The buyers then applied this pus to their penises, infecting themselves and allowing them to go on medical leave.

In Italy in the 16th century, it was common for the upper-class gentleman to hire a wetnurse for his wife and child. It was mutually understood between the mother, father and wetnurse that the wetnurse's job was to relieve the mother of some of the tensions of taking care of the child, as well as relieving the new father's sexual tensions.

In ancient Rome, baker's girls called aelicariae sold, among other things, bread rolls called colyphia. *Coliphia* was a slang term for "penis." These baker's girls often made extra money by selling themselves to their customers.

Another kind of working girl, the bustuariae, prostituted herself in cemeteries and added to her income by taking extra work as a paid mourner at funerals.

Japanese courtesans, called yuja, hooked their paying lovers by writing them love letters. The real selling point, however, was when the yuja included a lock of hair or clipping of a fingernail. Of course, the shy courtesan, having so many men to tempt, couldn't actually give up these parts of her body. Instead, she was supplied with these items by paid grave-robbers who took them off of corpses.

§

Prostitution has, in some times, been a feature of religious faith:

The ancient Cyprean parents sent their daughters away for a time before their marriage. They sent the girls to the coast so that they could prostitute themselves to the sailors. They did this to earn money for their marriage portion, and to give to Venus as an offering for their chastity after their marriage.

Herodotus, the Greek historian, noted that in Babylonia,

> Every woman who is a native of the country must once in her life go and sit in the temple there [the Temple of Mylitta] and give herself to a strange man. She is not allowed to go home until a man has thrown a silver coin into her lap and taken her outside to lie with him. The woman has no privilege of choice—she must go with the first man who throws her money. When she has lain with him, her duty to the goddess is discharged and she may go home.

The temple kept the silver coin, of course. The girl who had lost her virginity gave the coin to the temple, and on her way out made fun of the girls who had not been bedded yet. Consequently, after leaving the temple, every woman, no matter how virtuous, had slept with a man for money, not love. The more homely women often waited weeks before they were called upon.

§

Prostitution has long been considered an outlet to which men could go to preserve the purer women:

In ancient Rome, brothels were considered to be a necessary institution of society. Horace (65–8 B.C.) reasoned, "Young men, when their veins are full of gross lust, should drop in there, rather than grind some husband's private mill."

§

In the early 1800s in Algiers, whores bought monthly business licenses. In a city of 30,000 people, there were 3,000 whores registered. The local police, or mezonars, paid a fee to the government, with the extra money from licensing going to the mezonar as the collector of the fee. This profit encouraged the mezonar to create more prostitutes. He spied on married and unmarried women, and when he caught one in an illicit sexual affair, he put the woman's name in his whore's registry—forcing her to become a prostitute for life. Twice a year he threw public parties, forcing the women on his whore's list to show up and inviting the males of the city. This increased his income even more.

The low station of the common whore has even put her below the level of humanity:

In the 15th-century towns of France, whores were tolerated. But in some instances, they were treated as physically tainted women. In 1441 in Avignon, it was made law that the hookers must buy anything in the market that they had touched.

At times, the position of prostitutes has had some prestige:

In the sixth century, German prostitutes were protected from violence by the law. The fine for assault against a whore was six sous. The fine for an assault against other women was three sous.

Charles VII (1403–1461) set up the Grande Abbaye whorehouse in Toulouse under state protection. The city and the local university (a very good source of clients) shared in the profits of the whorehouse. The income of the state-funded whorehouse was so valuable, and Charles' protection was so complete, that he placed the royal coat of arms over the doorway.

In Zurich, Switzerland, during the 15th and 16th centuries, visiting ambassadors had the honor of dining with the mayor and prostitutes of the city.

In 1434, Emperor Sigismund (1368–1432) and his royal court visited Ulm, Germany. For his visit, the town council bought velvet gowns for all the city's whores. The route to the whorehouses was lit by torchlight for their guests' convenience.

When Charles V (1500–1558) visited Nuremburg, the city's tarts greeted him dressed only in flowers.

Prostitutes have often been required to distinguish themselves from "virtuous" women:

The South Carolina Waxsaws could distinguish prostitutes from the other tribeswomen because whores were required to wear their hair short. Prostitution was accepted, but it was a grave offense if the loose lady wore her hair long, as the other women did.

Ancient Roman emperor Justinian (483–565) required Rome's registered prostitutes to dye their hair either yellow or blue.

In the mid-15th century, under King Louis XI, France allowed prostitution but demanded that prostitutes not dress as extravagantly as the higher-class women. They could not wear fur, expensive jewelry, belts or long trains. In some places, the dress code was even more restrictive; the whore had to wear Hell's own color: red.

In 18th-century France, after the French Revolution, prostitutes wore a very revealing costume: a classical Greek robe of very light muslin material. Underneath this nearly transparent material, they wore a chemise and petticoats. With increased competition, the muslin became thinner and more transparent. The petticoats and chemise were replaced by flesh-colored tights. Again, competition in the sex trade became so fierce that the harlots revealed more. They took the body stocking off, wearing absolutely nothing under the filmy thin "toga."

In the 14th century, the prostitutes of the Grande Abbaye whorehouse in Toulouse protested the dress code that distinguished whores from the other women. They were required to wear a white nun's habit to identify them as prostitutes. Charles VI (1368–1422) agreed to abolish the dress code, and this angered the public, who took out their anger physically on the prostitutes. To fight this abuse, the hookers closed the doors to the whorehouse. The loss of income by neighboring merchants and loss of pleasure by the clients put pressure on Charles VII (1403–1461) to overturn the judgment. The whores' strike worked, and the dress restriction was once again lifted.

At times, a different costume had a positive effect for the hooker:

A woman's sandal dating from sixth-century B.C. Greece has a message stamped in reverse on the sole. When this prostitute walked, the sole left a message imprinted on the ground. It said, Follow Me.

Prostitutes in Venice during the Renaissance were allowed by the city to market themselves by going topless.

In ancient Rome, courtesans were not allowed to go through the streets other than on foot. Only noblewomen were allowed to be carried through the streets by their servants in litters. This order was not followed very closely, and some courtesans rode about in litters. These litters were covered with drapes, and very often the courtesan earned her money in the street by admitting a male into her litter.

In ancient Rome, a prostitute could be disallowed from practicing her trade if a customer complained that she had bad breath.

Mystery has been an important enticement on the part of prostitutes advertising themselves. But others have preferred the more direct approach:

In 13th-century Hangchow, China, the lowest class of whores was known as Yu Chi: wildfowl. They inhabited houses without windows. Instead, these houses were peppered with peepholes. Interested men could look through these peepholes and see these harlots lounging in obscene positions. Very often the most popular peepholes were those looking in on a whore in performance with a customer.

Eighteenth-century Japanese whores of the lowest order traveled lightly. These cheap whores did not keep a room to perform their services. Instead, they kept a rolled-up mat on their backs. Once they had a customer, they dropped it in an alley or hidden spot and had the customer then and there.

The best Greek prostitute, available in Corinth, cost as much as one talent, or over $1,000. The cheaper hookers, inmates of the 1,000-bed Temple of Venus, serviced sailors and other low-budget customers. Their price: one obol, or about one cent. The most miserable and unattractive hooker could expect to sell herself for two-tenths of a cent.

Love, sex and marriage were specialized functions in ancient Greece—which meant that wives did not necessarily provide the Greek man with all three:

Sex and the Greek man was explained by the Athenian statesman (384–322 B.C.) Demosthenes: "We marry women to have legitimate children and to have faithful guardians of our homes. We have concubines for our daily service and comfort, and courtesans for the enjoyment of love."

The courtesan was a one-man prostitute. She was well paid for her performance:

The Renaissance courtesan of Rome, Veronica Franco, was one of the most highly paid lovers of any time. The price of just one kiss from Veronica's lips was enough to pay a servant for six months.

The more common and less fortunate prostitute of the time was more poorly paid:

At the time of the Renaissance, in Nicaragua, sex with a prostitute cost 10 cocoa beans.

The price of a prostitute in Europe in 1420 was often less than the price of an egg.

The Greek hetaera, Lamina, sold her sexual services to the King of Macedon. He happily paid her fee, passing the expense on to his subjects. He taxed soap to raise Lamina's fee: 250 talents, or about $30,000.

Concubinage, the practice of taking a woman not as a full-fledged wife but merely for her sexual advantages, has been very popular at certain times in history:

In the late 11th century in England, the church began to demand that its servants become celibate and give up their wives. In 1129, the men of the church who did not maintain celibacy were punished. However, King Henry I saw his opportunity to increase his treasury. He taxed all holy men for the opportunity to keep a concubine.

Sexual offenses on the part of the clergy were up to 50 times higher, per capita, than those of the general population. By the 16th century, the clergy was considered the largest employer of the 100,000 English prostitutes practicing their trade.

Southern women in America of the 19th century who had black blood, however small an amount, had a dismal future. Women who were only one-eighth black were common. They were called quadroons. These women had few opportunities in life. It became almost custom to hold Quadroon Balls. These lavish balls featured well-mannered, beautiful quadroon girls accompanied by their mothers or aunts. Well-to-do white men attended these balls and assessed the girls. Then the interested man approached the girl's chaperone. In a very mannered way, he described how well he could keep the girl. Then he inquired as to the cost. These arrangements to take a girl from her mother as a mistress were very businesslike and polite.

Sailors visiting Tahiti in the 19th century could earn the affections of Tahitian girls by presenting them with nails from the hulls of their ships.

The free-love Tahitians did not have a concept of prostitution, so the girls merely considered the nails as gifts. However, there was a catch: the more beautiful a girl was, the longer nail she demanded. Once this became a custom, the girls' parents would present the sailors with a twig the length of a nail demanded for their daughter.

Prostitutes have not necessarily been poor, abandoned or wanton women:

The ancient Greeks had "religious prostitutes" who spent their time praying, educating themselves and soliciting men to earn money for their temples. The Greek, Anixeles, described the hetaera thusly: "The woman who speaks with reserve, and gives her favors to those who want to satisfy their natural need, is called an Hetaera, or 'good friend', for the sake of her friendship."

Because these women were very cultured, talented, highly intelligent and extremely attractive, they had far higher status than mere common prostitutes, or even other women. The hetaerae women were the first women in a male-dominated society to be considered the equal of men.

Sixteenth-century Italian courtesans had the same high status as their hetaera sisters. They used this status to pry political secrets out of high-ranking, loose-lipped clients, and passed the information on to the police.

Catherine de Médicis (1519–1589), queen of Henry II of France, organized the court ladies for political purposes. Between 200 and 300 of these well-bred, well-mannered women slept with politicians to keep the court informed of all plots and plans for and against the monarch. These women "rewarded" those loyal to the king and squeezed information out of the king's enemies. They were called the Queen's Flying Squadron.

In most cultures, the chief aim of associating with courtesans was sensual pleasure:

Courtesans in ancient China spent only a portion of their time as bedmates. The man who could afford a courtesan likely already had several wives and concubines, whom he was obligated to sexually satisfy.

The courtesan, then, was a woman with which the man could feel companionship. The personal association with courtesans was freer than that of husband and wife, so the girl for hire was treated as a person and less of a sex object than even the man's wife.

The romantic notion of medieval knights jousting for the honor of a smile from their lady love was quite different from the reality. Many times the lady they were trying to impress was a whore. A woman of lesser nobility often had to add to her husband's income. For this reason, the winner's purse from a jousting tournament often went to pay for the lady's sexual services—usually in a tent set up specifically for this purpose.

A prostitute did not necessarily have to capitalize on her feminine charms to excite interest:

In ancient Rome, some prostitutes made the most of their looks, while others attracted another type of customer—by dressing like young boys.

The brothel in Pompeii, when receiving a new girl, a virgin, held an auction for the pleasure of her favors. The lucky bidder was allowed to have her the whole night.

The concept of having temple prostitutes originated with the ancient Greeks. It was revived in a modified form:

After the end of the Holy Crusades, whores who earned their keep by traveling with the Crusaders returned to do what they did best. Although the townspeople made good use of the women, they objected to their high profile.

In 1347 in the papal city of Avignon, France, a brothel was set up. It was sponsored by the Catholic Church under the patronage of Joanna of Naples. The prostitutes divided their time between prayer, religious study, strict attendance of services and bedding down with customers. Only Christians could be serviced by these holy whores. Jews were especially unwelcome. The money earned from their erotic duties went to the Catholic Church. Pope Julius II was so enthusiastic about the worship-whorship arrangement that in the early 16th century he opened his own church-brothel in the Vatican City.

Prostitution has been carefully regulated at times—and even mannerly at other times:

In 15th-century France, prostitutes were not allowed to accept just any kind of customer. They could not accept very young men. They could not take in two people who were related at the same time. The harlots could not sleep with married men who came from their hometown. The prostitutes also had intercourse in no other way but the traditional male-superior position. Intercourse was performed in much the same way as marital intercourse.

If the church couldn't or didn't want to regulate or abolish prostitution, it could keep its sense of humor about it:

It is unclear how concerned about prostitution Cardinal Hugo was, considering how rampant it was in his hometown of Lyons, France, in 1251. As he said farewell to the city after a term of eight years, he remarked: "When we first came here, there were three or four brothels. We leave behind us but one. I must confess, however, that it extends without interruption from the eastern gate to the western gate."

Licensed prostitution has been a common feature of many societies:

Houses of pleasure in China during the T'ang dynasty had their own trade association and paid taxes. Their status was the same as any other business. Both the whores and house owners had rights under licensing. On the one hand, a girl was obligated to perform as per her contract and could be held liable for breaking it. On the other hand, girls had the right to expose an unfair brothel owner. A lower class of hookers had no rights, as they were unlicensed and thus unprotected.

Fortunate whores could dramatically increase their business if they could find a large clientele in a festive mood:

It was believed for a very long time that married women were forbidden to travel to Corinth to see the Olympics in ancient Greece, because the athletes performed in the nude. However, unmarried girls were allowed to view the sports, and the nude body was not an unusual sight in everyday Greece. Considering Corinth's very healthy trade in sex, it is more likely that the Olympics was a good opportunity for men to indulge in extramarital sex.

In Constance, Germany, a council of the church was held from 1414 to 1418. This event drew a great number of out-of-towners, including

1,400 whores. No complaints were made by the citizens or churchmen, as the council officials and others used their services regularly. One of the hundreds of harlots kept herself so busy at this conference that she was allowed to retire in luxury afterward.

One of the best business opportunities whores in ancient Rome could find was among the traffic of the Roman spectators exiting the Circus Maximus after the suggestive or outright dirty comedies offered, or after the brutal and sadistic gladiatorial battles, sacrifices and animal fights had stirred their blood.
   Often the prostitutes did not even wait for the end of the public spectacles. They joined the crowd in the Circus Maximus, and often the inflamed the passions of the spectators demanded instant gratification. It was then that the whore took her customer to have sex in the arched fornices under the seats of the Circus Maximus.

Prostitutes have not been the only beneficiaries of the sexually curious:

In Cabul, Afghanistan, in the 19th century, a particularly seedy district included the Street of Fornication. On the Street of Fornication was every kind of erotic entertainment and service. This theme drew many tourists innocent of the ways of this street. Among the vendors were those selling sugar-coated cakes. It was only after it was too late that the out-of-town rube tourist realized that what he had paid for was sugar-coated goat dung.

With organized prostitution, the red-light districts could become very well integrated into the city:

About 1276 in London, a red-light district came into existence. The area was boldly named Gropecuntlane, which contained streets named Codpiece Lane, Shitburnelane and Slut's Hole.

Among the more colorful names for brothels was the Cardinal's Cap. This was a reference to the cap worn in Roman-Greek times by the holy men of the Cult of Priapus. As its name indicates, the Cult of Priapus worshiped the phallus. The cap worn by the holy men was red, with folds resembling those of the male foreskin. These caps became very popular and were worn by many of London's tradesmen of the time, until the city's lawmakers outlawed them as being obscene.

In ancient Rome, cheaply bought whores had sex with their customers wherever they could. It became habit for them to do their business in fornices—short arches a few feet high, on the sides of buildings. It was from this familiar place for illicit sex that the word *fornicate* derived.

Red-light districts have been popular areas for thousands of years:

During the Chinese T'ang dynasty, in Yangchow, there existed a particularly large red-light district. Blue two-story houses, on both sides of the streets, greeted the erotic adventurer. These houses were the dwellings of jade girls—high-class prostitutes. The line of blue houses stretched unbroken for four miles.

The late 1800s saw a great increase in foreign traffic into Japan. A major seaport 300 miles from Hong Kong was Amoy. This busy center had 300,000 people. Because of the high commercial traffic, there was one whorehouse for every 82 people, and 50,000 girls, or half of all females in that city, worked as prostitutes.

In the late 1700s in London, a businesswoman by the name of Miss Fawkland ambitiously rented three St. James Street houses. These she called the Temples of Aurora, Flora and Mystery. The client entered through Aurora. It housed a dozen girls between the ages of 11 and 16. In this palace of pleasure, the girls were taught the mysteries of sex. The Temple of Flora contained 150 young women, among them graduates of Aurora. The Temple of Mystery specialized in servicing the most sexually depraved and hardened customers. These women were so jaded, they were not allowed to associate with the girls from the other two temples.

Whorehouses in Berlin were subject to a regulation in 1792 that prohibited alcohol in whorehouses. This rule was created because liquors were "great inducements to debauchery."

Armies have recognized the needs of its soldiers and often provided extracurricular activity for its recruits:

In 1269 Louis IX left France to lead his men on the Crusades. Before he left, he proclaimed that all whorehouses were to be destroyed. This caused problems for some whores, but others responded to the order by joining the Crusaders as camp whores. A large number of homeless hookers followed Louis IX all the way to the seaport of Aigues-Mortes.

A great many even set sail with the soldiers, following them to Jerusalem. The result of Louis IX's order, then, was merely to encourage more whores to follow the Crusaders to their Holy War.

The Chinese Ming dynasty (1368–1644) was the age of the first real military bordello. These military whorehouses were located at spots along the 1,400-mile-long Great Wall of China. The military whores, Ying-chi, in addition to servicing the soldiers, trained reserve soldiers and helped defend the walls against the Mongols.

During World War I, Germany had traveling brothels. The madam and her girls followed the progress of the German army, staying just behind the lines. Seen as a necessity to keep morale high, the German high command fully endorsed the troop of trollops.

Customers were checked thoroughly for disease, and condoms were dispensed by the medical corps. The corps also collected the fees. Each man was allotted one half hour, unless the rush for the women's services was great. If so, each soldier was given 10 minutes with a girl before the sergeant declared him finished—whether he truly was or not.

At the end of World War I, military brothels did not disappear. The occupying Allied forces' sexual needs were taken care of, with the bill being picked up by the defeated German nation. With the Germans paying, these whorehouses were lavish and numerous. In the Rhine alone, there were 19 brothels in 16 communities. The average German whore received anywhere from 60 to 100 men a day.

Venereal disease has always been a risk when sex has been sold:

In the autumn of 1494, Neapolitan and Spanish soldiers set up quarters in the Italian cities of Florence, Rome and Siena. These soldiers and their company of whores made merry in Rome over the winter. By the spring of 1495, syphilis was rampant. The outbreak of venereal disease was so widespread that only the great outbreak of the Plague rivaled it. Across Europe in 1495, a full 5 percent of the population died of the ugly syphilis disease. Eventually, 30 percent of Europe at that time would die of it. Many thousands died slow, agonizing deaths. Those who didn't die of syphilis were often killed by physicians who performed painful and disgusting experiments in a vain attempt to cure the disease.

The powerlessness of all to remedy or even control the disease only made the population more fatalistic and anxious to get whatever pleasures they could, while they were still alive. Although people died in droves, the birth rate actually increased. A panicked population became amoral, and every kind of public chaos and crime occurred, especially those of the sexual sort.

Japanese prostitutes in the Meiji period of the late 1800s played party games in the brothels to arouse their customers. A common game was Fukagawa-Asagawa. In this game, geisha girls danced, slowly raising their kimonos up as the "river" got higher. Gradually, the girls briefly exposed their vaginas—then covered them up with their fans.

A variation of this party game was Chonkina. The girls danced around singing, "Chonkina...chonkina...HAI!" The last girl to yell "Hai" had to remove a piece of clothing until a girl had lost all of her clothes. Then the rest of the girls stripped down.

Prostitutes did not always earn their way by intercourse:

London of the mid-1600s hosted a society of Dutch whores. The organization was called the Half-Crown Chuck Office. These women earned their way by standing on their heads and spreading their legs wide, enticing men to deposit, or "chuck" in, half crowns into their vaginas.

In many other cases, women were forced into the role of prostitute completely against their will:

The cheapest Chinese brothels employed slaves of one kind or another: female prisoners of war, female criminals, and women whose relatives were prosecuted for crimes, whose punishment included the prostitution of a female relative. These women were forced to make money for the government brothels, while receiving only enough to stay alive.

The men of the Kambaramba tribe in the central Amazon area were poor hunters and bad warriors and could keep no land. To survive, whenever hungry or threatened by another tribe, the Kambaramba men sold their women. Any female 12 or older was sold in exchange for food or given away to please a threatening rival tribe.

With the massive immigration of Europeans to Japan in the late 1800s came greater opportunities for the whore to make money. However, many Japanese whores and brothelkeepers refused to service Europeans.

They considered sex with Europeans to be disgusting, calling the new-comers ketto—"the hairy barbarians." Some whores killed themselves rather than have the brothel owner force a European on them.

On the Line Islands, when a man married, he married all his wife's sisters as well. If he did not want responsibility for any or all of the sisters, they were simply obligated to become prostitutes.

About 1490 in Paris, Jean Tisserand opened a home for wayward girls to allow them to stop working the streets for their bread. It was called Refuge des Filles penitentes.

Unfortunately, many poor girls who were very poor but not prostitutes sold themselves only in order to gain entrance to this comfortable "orphanage." This increased, not decreased, the population of Paris whores.

The New Hollanders were tolerant of prostitutes. This very primitive tribe performed delicate surgery—removing the ovaries of women. The only women whose ovaries were removed, however, were the tribe's prostitutes.

On the Arizona border, a tribe called the Sinaloa initiated new prostitutes at a large festival. After this initiation, all the women of the tribe were obliged to serve any and all who met the price. Not even marriage could excuse the girl from the obligation to satisfy the man who could pay the going rate for her company.

During the Middle Ages in England, a woman guilty of being a whore was set on a ducking-stool. This was a chair at the end of a pole. The prostitute was tied to the chair. Several men lifted the pole and dunked her into a slimy, stinking pond three times.

About A.D. 100 the Teutons punished prostitutes by disemboweling them or suffocating them in excrement.

The sexual favors of a wife have not always been jealously guarded by the husband who could profit by it:

Tahitian tribal chiefs paid their male servants by allowing them, on occasion, to sleep with their wives. The chiefs had no shortage of help around their households, with such spectacular compensation offered.

Among the Marquesans, the king's servants were allowed to have sex with his wives. While he decided when and with whom, he was always conscious of the fact that the help had to be satisfied, or they would leave his household.

Many men have sold their sexuality. Throughout history, hundreds of thousands of men have been castrated for the sake of employment:

In a city called Messelaumeeyeh in Khartoum, in the district of Darfour, there existed a eunuchry. It was called Dewwausheh and it was the world's greatest source of eunuchs. Sudani boys between the ages of 4 and 10 were captured and taken there. But for every eunuch who left Dewwausheh, taken to Khartoum to be sold, 10 died, not having recovered from the surgery. It was estimated that nearly 30,000 boys died each year to supply 3,000 eunuchs annually.

In most countries where harems existed, the only males allowed around the women were eunuchs. There were severe penalties for the uncastrated man found among a man's harem:

In Persia, it was a serious offense for an outsider to be caught in a man's gynaeceum, or "harem-room." For violating a man's personal stable of mates, the punishment was merciless. The fugitive was stripped down and given to grooms and slaves, to be used to satisfy their homosexual needs.

At one time, Chinese eunuchs wore their pickled testicles around their necks.

It was not until the 20th century that eunuchry was totally dismantled:

As late as the 1930s in China, there lived eunuchs. The last reminder of this strange and sad occupation was a building that housed former servants of the Imperial Palace. The name of the boardinghouse: Refuge for Distressed Eunuchs.

STRANGE SEXUAL OCCURRENCES

FEMALE DEFORMITIES

STRANGE MEDICAL QUIRKS CONCERNING BREASTS

Dr. Raoul Leroy of the Ville-Eurard Asylum met a strange woman. This 23-year-old patient, mentally disturbed, had produced milk from her breast since 10 years of age.

In Rome in 1671, a woman was put on public display as a medical freak. The woman had four breasts, each capable of producing milk.

In Capetown, South Africa, Gardner reported seeing a six-breasted negress. All breasts produced milk.

In 1886 the Imperial Academy of Vienna heard a presentation by Neugebauer. He claimed to have seen a woman with 10 breasts and produced a picture to verify his claim. Some of these breasts, however, consisted of only a nipple and a areola.

UNUSUAL VARIATIONS IN FEMALE SEXUAL ORGANS

Bartholin saw a woman whose pubic hair was so long, she braided it.

Jahn saw a woman whose pubic hair reached down to her knees.

A woman in ancient Rome, according to Colombo, had a clitoris as long as a person's little finger. The clitoris hardened and eventually broke off.

Otto of Breslau reported a clitoris that measured four and one-half inches long and one and one-half inches in transverse diameter. It belonged to an African woman, and it plainly projected from her vulva. While relaxed, it covered the vaginal orifice completely.

A 20-year-old Russian peasant woman was admitted into a Russian hospital after her husband's first attempts at lovemaking were painful and left her, technically, a virgin.

Upon examination, it was found that she possessed a tough hymen, with an opening just large enough to allow a little finger. Beyond her hymen was yet another hymen. Both hymens were surgically broken, and coitus was then possible.

Glasgow, England's Dr. Saint Clair related the cases of two of his patients. One was a 30-year-old woman, married 10 years, whose hymen was perfectly intact despite her husband's best efforts. It was strong and elastic and, except for a tiny opening, completely blocked entry.

Another patient had been married for 21 years and was 43 years old. She had the hymen of a virgin, unruptured in spite of regular intercourse.

Taylor had seen prostitutes who had been in the trade for between 7 and 11 years, who had still retained their hymens.

Martinelli witnessed a 30-year-old woman giving birth, her baby pressing against her perfectly closed hymen, while the child was on its way into this world.

A Strasberg physician, Stoltz, had a case of a woman keeping her perforated, but not destroyed, hymen—even after having given birth. It had taken the appearance of a slack diaphragm after the first birth, but was finally destroyed with the birth of her second child.

Payne related the case of a 35-year-old woman who was apparently of good health. She had been in labor for 36 hours when doctors discovered she had no vaginal opening. Instead, the head of her child appeared from her anus. It was removed with no complications. The woman and her husband had found anal sex to be natural and seemed unconcerned about her lack of a vaginal opening.

Dr. Robb from Johns Hopkins Hospital detailed a case of a 20-year-old woman. She was found to have a double vagina.

Vallisneri interviewed a woman who had two uteri. The first opened into the vagina, the second led into the rectum.

In 1734, Louis, a French surgeon, had a patient who had no exterior genitals. She had her sexual tract ending internally in the lower end of the alimentary canal.

An 18-year-old prostitute was examined who claimed that she had never menstruated. Her outer organs were normally formed, but she had no vagina, uterus or ovaries. Her sexual partners were satisfied by penetration of the urethra, which had been enlarged.

MALE SEXUAL DEFORMITIES

MALES WITH UNUSUAL BREAST CONFIGURATIONS

Jean Benoit Erandellius documented the situation of a nine-year-old boy. The boy, a beggar, had a chest slightly smaller than average. But when he squeezed his breasts together, milk was drawn from them.

In 1894 a 24-year-old army wagon driver was treated for an abscess. While in the Val-de-Grace Hospital in Paris, he was brought to the attention of Dr. Renauldin. Upon examination, the doctor found this otherwise masculine man to have unmistakably female breasts.

Dr. Steinborn of Thorn treated a case of an extra breast growing on the thigh. The patient was a father of 12. For six years, the breast had been growing on his right inner thigh. When examined by the doctor, it was found to be the size of a goose egg. It was soft but firm, and had an areola.

An issue of the *Gazette Medicale* in Paris, dated 1835, had a report on the case of a 21-year-old Parisian male. His scrotum was enlarged and had the texture of a female breast. Part of it was even pink-colored. Milk was being secreted from the young man's scrotum.

ANOMALIES OF THE MALE SEXUAL ORGANS

While with the British Medical Corps, Dr. Sundaresa Ayzer examined a 19-year-old boy with a curious deformity. This boy was a native of Trichinopoly. He possessed a normal penis but had three testicles. The extra testicle was positioned above his left testicle.

French physicians encountered a strange condition they named penis palme. In this condition, the penis and testicles were not separate but shared a common skin. Understandably, erection was very painful for sufferers of penis palme.

In Naples, Italy, one Dr. Bruni witnessed a case of multiple genitals. The patient possessed two separate members, each of nearly average size. He also had a second anus. Underneath each penis hung a single testicle.

Antonio de Ramos of Novo Mindello, an eight-year-old boy, was discovered by physicians in 1865. His face was boyish, but his hips, like those of a female, were wider than his shoulders. His penis was normal in form and size. He had no testicles, but rather something of a vagina with distinct labia and scent. He urinated through both organs, but more frequently from the vagina.

CURIOUS MENSTRUAL ABERRATIONS

One girl had her first menstruation at 15 years of age. It was not until six months later that she had her second menstruation. It lasted three weeks, without stopping. She had since menstruated only twice a year, in March and September, for three weeks each time.

Sophie Gentz, a little Jewish girl, was reported by Warner as having started menstruating at the age of 23 months. Her period occurred regularly and unceasingly from that point onward.

One girl complained that she had no menstrual flow, even though she was old enough and healthy enough to have started menstruating. She felt the emotional and physical symptoms, and then would experience an itchiness on the tip of her right index finger. To stop the itching, she would rub her finger vigorously enough to break a blood vessel. After losing about two ounces of blood, the bleeding would stop. Then, the general symptoms of menstruation, aches and tiredness, would disappear.

In 1890 a 37-year-old woman underwent surgery to relieve an inflammation of the womb. In 1894, the woman began to feel the symptoms of having her period. Her thumb began to redden four days after the feelings of discomfort. Then a small stream of blood flowed from the thumb, and kept slowly flowing for five days. This experience occurred for five days every month, starting on the 28th day of each month.

A young girl was referred to Dr. Lermoyez in 1899. She complained that she bled through her right ear monthly. She had been menstruating through her ear for three years. Later, only every second or third period occurred through the ear, the other instances occurring through the normal method.

In London, England, a Dr. Barnes observed a girl who menstruated through her nipples.

There was reported an instance of a girl who had a curious side effect from the appearance of her period. During the days she menstruated, she was stone-deaf.

One unfortunate girl was known to have gone blind for no apparent reason—until the blindness ceased with the start of her first period.

A 15-year-old girl was said to have suffered in a most unusual way during her period. The young girl constantly felt the need to turn somersaults during the time she menstruated.

A guardian of a local estate visited a student of surgery, a certain M. Caestryck Jr. The man was in good health, except for a periodic bleeding from his nose. Caestryck had bled monthly since the age of 16. On average, his "period" yielded about one and a half quarts of blood.

One man, beginning in puberty, experienced swelling and sensitivity around his nipple. The feeling was accompanied by erotic dreams and sexual stimulation. This occurred every 28 days and lasted about two days.

In Roche-Calais, France, on June 24, 1756, a Dr. Leboeuf was called to an accident. A shepherd had injured his breastbone in a fall. Leboeuf was going to "bleed" the patient, but the mistress of the house advised against it, as "the young man was having his period."

Leboeuf, upon seeing the patient, assumed it was a woman in men's clothing. The mistress confirmed that the patient was a male. But this man had been menstruating through his penis. These periods lasted two days, often yielding as much as four ounces of blood. His penis was normal and healthy in all other respects. The young man was one of 16 boys in the family. He also had a perfectly normal sister. All his brothers suffered from this female characteristic, as did his father.

A man of good heredity and good health began from puberty to experience congestion in his penis and testicles, had erotic thoughts and began to menstruate two or three days every month through his penis. At the age of 45, menstruation ceased.

UNUSUAL INSTANCES OF EARLY MATURITY

The *Journal de Medicine* reported on a patient of Dr. Fages de Chazelles. The patient was a child, a resident of Cahors. He was physically mature, though only four years old. At this young age, he had a sexual appetite and actively pursued women.

An English child was observed by physicians as having advanced maturity. At the age of three years and one month, the boy was 3 feet, 11 inches tall. His penis while flaccid was three inches long, and erect, it was four and one-third inches long. He had a substantial growth of pubic hair, a very masculine voice, and the strength of a nine-year-old. He also had the intelligence of a six-year-old.

A child in Falaise, Normandy, was recognized by the Histoire de l'Academie des Sciences as having a very rare condition. The six-month-old child showed all the signs of puberty.

The Duke de Roquelaure fathered a child who was born less than six months after conception.

A 35-year-old woman was due to give birth in April 1883. In May of that year, she had labor pains that quickly subsided. Over several months, she experienced the same early signs of impending childbirth. By September of 1883, the womb had dilated, the baby still waiting to be born. Its movements became excruciating for the mother. Finally, on November 6, 1883, she gave birth. The 13-pound child was born after a pregnancy lasting 476 days.

A Strasburg, Germany, woman, Anne Vivier, gave birth to a son on April 30, 1748. On September 16, 1748, four and a half months later, she again gave birth. The second child, a daughter, did not appear to be premature. She was a fully developed newborn.

Kimura witnessed a strange case of abnormal childbirth. A Japanese woman's pregnancy appeared normal. But one day the arm of the fetus was seen pressing against the inside of the woman's skin, just above her navel. An incision was made and the fetus removed. The baby had gestated outside the womb.

A church register in Derbyshire, England, from 1650 reads thusly:

> "April ye 20, 1650, was buried Emme, the wife of Thomas Toplace, who was found delivered of a child after she had lain two hours in the grave."

Dr. Saviad in 1686 performed an autopsy on a woman who had died during childbirth. Examination of the dead woman revealed a fossilized fetus in her left ovary. Another fetus was found in a hollow between the womb and the rectum, near her sacral arch.

A native woman in Peru was struck by lightning. The next day, the deceased pregnant woman's abdomen was ordered to be opened. A living child was removed from the deceased woman's womb.

After experiencing a terrible pain in the abdomen and a hemorrhage, a woman felt the urgent need to relieve her bowels. After the feeling passed, the woman thought about it no further. Again she felt the extreme pain and the need to go to the bathroom. She passed a quantity of blood and felt a large blockage. In seeking to remove it, she grabbed the leg of her fetus. She was rushed to a hospital, where a fetus measuring nine inches was removed from her anus.

A healthy, normal 11-year-old girl began to feel a swelling in the abdomen. McIntyre reported that the abdomen expanded at the rate of one and one-half inches a day. After 10 days, surgery was performed on the right side of the abdomen. A five-pound fetus was removed.

In 1944, Miss Emmie Marie Jones collapsed, suffering from shock and severe exhaustion. After nine months, a daughter was born. She claimed to have been a virgin. This claim was supported by the fact that the daughter grew up to be an identical twin to her mother.

An ovarian tumor was removed from the body of a 16-year-old girl. The tumor contained live eggs and sperm, although the physical evidence revealed her to be a virgin.

A grown man, according to Ruysch, carried a tumor around for several years before he finally required surgery to remove it. When he was finally operated on, the growth in the man's abdomen was found to be a lump of hair, molar teeth and other parts of a fetus.

A surgeon, Dr. Velpeau, in an operation witnessed by 500 medical students and hospital staff, retrieved an embryo from a man's body. The operation, undertaken at the Hopital de la Charite in Paris, was a success. The doctor pulled ribs, vertebrae and other parts of a fetus from the patient's scrotum.

The Royal Society of London received a report by Huxham in 1748. In it he described the incidence of a newborn carrying another child. The second child was an embryo found in the infant's anus.

A Pomeranian woman became pregnant three times. These three pregnancies yielded a total of 11 children. She produced two sets of quadruplets and a set of triplets.

William Stratton of Paddington, England, died in 1734 at the ripe old age of 97. During his life he fathered 28 children by his first wife, and 17 by his second—a total of 45 children.

In 1852 a woman gave birth to her last set of triplets. This last set of triplets was her eighth. All 24 children born to the woman, married nine years, were daughters.

Mrs. Marie Austin, of Washington, D.C., was married 30 years. During that time, until her death in 1882 at the age of 60, she gave birth to 44 children. Every one of them was male.

A patient of Dr. Vassali of Lugano was a day-worker near Rome. Flavia Granata had 62 children in 26 years. She had a total of 41 daughters and 21 sons.

Her first child was a daughter. She then had sextuplets, all boys. She then gave birth to male quintuplets. A set of triplets added three daughters to the family. Following them were several sets of twins. Her last pregnancy yielded four boys.

A Dr. Marcel Beaudouin related a case of a Russian peasant. The man, named Wasilef, was twice married. His second wife yielded two sets of triplets and six pairs of twins. His first wife gave birth to four sets of quadruplets, seven sets of triplets, and 16 pairs of twins. Wasilef fathered a total of 87 children.

John Gilley was born in Ireland in 1690 and died in Augusta, Maine, in 1813 at the age of 123. In 1750 he emigrated to the United States, and 15 years later, at the age of 75, gave up his bachelorhood. He and his 18-year-old wife had eight children. His wife, understandably, survived him. She claimed that her husband was sexually active until the age of 120.

Joseph Surrington was born in 1637 and died 160 years later, in 1797. He left a widow, who was the last of several wives, and several offspring. At the time of his death, his oldest child was 103 years old. The youngest, born when Surrington was 151 years old, was only 9 years old.